# MRCP Part 2
# Best of Five Practice Questions

MRCP Part 2

# Best of Five Practice Questions

WITH EXPLANATORY ANSWERS

**SHIBLEY RAHMAN**
MA MB BChir PhD (all Cantab) MRCP(UK) LLB (Hons)
British Lung Foundation

*and*

**AVINASH SHARMA**
MBBS MRCP(UK)
Consultant Physician
Luton & Dunstable Hospital NHS Foundation Trust

Radcliffe Publishing
Oxford • New York

**Radcliffe Publishing Ltd**
18 Marcham Road
Abingdon
Oxon OX14 1AA
United Kingdom

**www.radcliffe-oxford.com**

Electronic catalogue and worldwide online ordering facility.



British Library Cataloguing in Publication Data

A catalogue record for this book is available from the British Library.

ISBN-13: 978 184619 360 6

The paper used for the text pages of this book is FSC certified. FSC (The Forest Stewardship Council) is an international network to promote responsible management of the world's forests.

Typeset by Pindar NZ, Auckland, New Zealand
Printed and bound by TJI Digital, Padstow, Cornwall, UK

# Contents

Preface vii
About the authors x
Some normal values xi

1 Cardiology 1
Questions 2
Answers 12
Learning Points 16

2 Haematology, oncology and immunology 17
Questions 20
Answers 39
Learning Points 45

3 Dermatology 49
Questions 50
Answers 52

4 Infectious diseases and tropical medicine 55
Questions 56
Answers 81
Learning Points 88

5 Rheumatology 89
Questions 90
Answers 98
Learning Points 102

6 Clinical pharmacology and toxicology 103
Questions 104
Answers 119
Learning Points 124

7 Gastroenterology and hepatology 127
Questions 128
Answers 144
Learning Points 148

8 Respiratory medicine 149
Questions 150
Answers 168
Learning Points 174

9 Nephrology 175
Questions 176
Answers 212
Learning Points 229

10 Neurology, ophthalmology and psychiatry 233
Questions 234
Answers 269
Learning Points 279

11 Endocrinology and metabolic medicine 281
Questions 283
Answers 308
Learning Points 317

Index 319

# Preface

The Royal College of Physicians have developed an examination, which they intend to be fair and to be an appropriate test of postgraduate knowledge in doctors preparing for higher specialist training. The academic aims are stated clearly:

- to test a wide range of up-to-date medical knowledge so that physicians in training are encouraged to develop their full clinical and professional potential
- to maintain and improve the practice of clinical medicine
- to provide a sound basis for continuing medical education.

Preparation for the examination is intended to encourage physicians in training to acquire relevant knowledge and understanding. Their examination, and this series of books, utilises the one from five, or '*best of five*' question format, and the aim of this format is to assess 'seasoned' doctors' knowledge and clinical experience.

These books intend to reflect some of the 'favourite topics' which have become recurrent in the examination, and therefore put special emphasis on those topics which are more likely to appear in the MRCP examination. The examination itself is very carefully set, and the pass mark depends very much on a pre-determined standard. That said, if a question proves to be too difficult or too easy, it may not be included in the final set of questions used to determine a candidate's pass. Likewise, there is usually a set of 'target' questions that is used to make sure that the standard of the examination remains the same across all sittings. The length of each chapter reflects the weighting given to each of the subjects. Each chapter follows exactly the same format (except for one): Questions, Answers and Learning points (designed to include crucial information in relation to each subject).

We have structured the book so that it is very much a manual with which to learn, rather than for you to feel examined from the word go. For that purpose, we have tried as hard as possible to provide explanations for why the correct answers are correct, as well as some guidance on why the incorrect answers are incorrect.

The answers are therefore comprehensive and focus on the fundamental principles of medical practice. Learning points are provided for some topics, to add further interest. The number of questions in each subject category by and large reflects the weightings of the actual examination, rather than the interests of the authors. The questions are arranged by subject area, so that structured revision may take place, and junior doctors who are potential candidates for the examination can focus on particular areas where they may feel that they have had little clinical experience, such as, for example, neurology.

The primary intention of this book is to assist people who have passed Part 1 to accomplish Part 2 successfully. The questions reflect to some extent those topics that are not covered as much in Part 2 as they are in Part 1, as well as covering comprehensively those topics common to both. Consequently, we hope that this book may be useful to candidates of both Part 1 and Part 2. Specifically, whilst there is no category for statistics, epidemiology and evidence-based medicine in Part 2 (unlike Part 1), it is expected that some questions will reflect these topics.

The MRCP(UK) examination has become in itself a 'gold standard' in terms of being a nationally and internationally sought-after qualification, and so attempting to reflect the quality of questions of the examination in this book has been difficult, as the wording of the questions that comprise the papers in real life are subject to intense scrutiny by various members of specialist groups. The aims, as outlined in the 'Part 1 syllabus', are to test a wide range of up-to-date medical knowledge, to maintain and improve the practice of clinical medicine, and to provide a sound basis for continuing medical education. As these are stated aims, it can be useful to look at recent taskforces within the Royal College of Physicians, developments from the General Medical Council, and the National Institute for Health and Clinical Excellence (NICE) guidelines published on the NICE website (*see* below). The latest information regarding the examination is available from the MRCP website – www.mrcpuk.org. Useful other clinical information can be obtained from the NICE website – www.nice.org.uk and the RCP website – www.rcplondon.ac.uk. The authors are especially grateful to the chapter reviewers for ensuring that the answers are consistent with up-to-date guidelines at the time of publication.

The marking system for the examination is straightforward. One mark (+1) is awarded for each correct answer:

- a correct answer to a *one from five* question
- a correct answer to an item in an *'n' from many* question.

Marks will not be awarded for answers in excess of the number required, or where the answer sheet is spoiled and unreadable by the optical marking scanner.

The MRCP(UK) Part 2 Written Examination is criterion-referenced, such that a candidate's performance is assessed in relation to an external standard of performance (pass mark) set by the examiners. The pass mark will be agreed for the examination as a whole and any candidate achieving this mark will pass.

There are three sittings per year of the Part 2 Written Examination. The authors draw your attention to the need to look up the current format of the examination on the MRCP website.

As of November 2008, the advice given was:

> The MRCP(UK) Part 2 Written Examination has a three-paper format. All Papers in the MRCP(UK) Part 2 Written Examination contain up to 100 multiple choice questions. The questions will usually have a clinical scenario, may include the results of investigations and may be illustrated.

Normal values for all chapters are included at the front of this book (subject-specific values are given in each chapter, as relevant). Whereas the exam will have these normal values in the actual question, we have included these values as separate tables so that you can get a good feel for them, as in real life!

We are most grateful to reviewers who carefully analysed both the questions and the answers, especially in light of the current evidence base. They include Dr Alexander Brand (Chelsea and Westminster Foundation NHS Trust), Dr Julian Collinson (Chelsea and Westminster NHS Foundation Trust), Dr Ameet Dhar (Imperial College Healthcare NHS Trust), Dr Jake Dunning (Chelsea and Westminster Foundation NHS Trust), Dr Dilys Lai (Chelsea and Westminster NHS Foundation Trust), Dr Daniel Patterson (University College Hospital London Foundation Trust), Dr Yohan Samarsinghe (West Middlesex NHS Trust), Dr Paul Warwicker (East and North Hertfordshire NHS Trust), and Dr Phil Wilkinson (East and North Hertfordshire Trust).

A final note: whilst the authors take full responsibility for the scientific material in this book, they do not take responsibility for drug dosages. These should be checked with an up-to-date copy of an appropriate reference source such as the *British National Formulary*.

Good luck!

**Dr S Rahman**
**Dr A Sharma**
***August 2009***

# About the authors

**Dr Shibley Rahman MA MB BChir PhD (all Cantab) MRCP(UK) LLB (Hons)** works as a Researcher for the British Lung Foundation, given his interests in evidence-based medicine and scientific communication to the public. He graduated in medicine from Cambridge in 2001, and attained his MRCP in 2005. He completed his research doctorate from Cambridge in the diagnosis and treatment of early onset dementias, and also has done post-doctoral research in the effect of visual cues in Parkinson's disease at the Institute of Neurology, Queen Square, London. He has written an extensive range of publications in both subject areas. Dr Rahman has a further academic interest in English law, particularly medical law and neuro-ethics. He was awarded his LLB (Hons) from BPP Law School, London in March 2009.

**Dr Avinash Sharma MBBS MRCP(UK)** is a Consultant Physician at the Luton & Dunstable Hospital NHS Foundation Trust. He trained in General and Geriatric Medicine from NW Thames (London) Deanery, after attaining his MRCP in the year 2003. His clinical and research interest focuses on understanding the patho-physiology and management of varied illnesses in the elderly population, with a special emphasis on Parkinson's disease, development of falls prevention and supported early discharge strategies. He has a keen interest in the training of medical students and junior doctors, and previously has helped in organising the final MB and MRCP PACES exams, while doing his higher specialist training at the Chelsea and Westminster Foundation NHS Trust in London.

# Some normal values

(Other normal values are given in the relevant chapter.)

**Haematology**

**Full blood count**

| | |
|---|---|
| haemoglobin (males) | 13.0–18.0 g/L |
| haemoglobin (females) | 11.5–16.5 g/L |
| haematocrit (males) | 0.40–0.52 |
| haematocrit (females) | 0.36–0.47 |
| MCV | 80–96 fL |
| MCH | 28–32 pg |
| MCHC | 32–35 g/L |
| white cell count | 4 –11 × $10^9$/L |
| white cell differential: | |
| neutrophils | 1.5–7 × $10^9$/L |
| lymphocytes | 1.5–4 × $10^9$/L |
| monocytes | 0–0.8 × $10^9$/L |
| eosinophils | 0.04–0.4 × $10^9$/L |
| basophils | 0–0.1 × $10^9$/L |
| platelet count | 150–400 × $10^9$/L |
| reticulocyte count | 25–85 × 109/L OR 0.5–2.4% |
| erythrocyte sedimentation rate (Westergren): | |
| Under 50 years: | |
| males | 0–15 mm/1st hr |
| females | 0–20 mm/1st hr |
| Over 50 years: | |
| males | 0–20 mm/1st hr |

| | |
|---|---|
| females | 0–30 mm/1st hr |
| **Chemistry** | |
| serum sodium | 137–144 mmol/L |
| serum potassium | 3.5–4.9 mmol/L |
| serum chloride | 95–107 mmol/L |
| serum bicarbonate | 20–28 mmol/L |
| anion gap | 12–16 mmol/L |
| serum osmolality | 275–295 mOsm/kg |
| serum urea | 2.5–7.5 mmol/L |
| serum creatinine | 60–110 μmol/L |
| serum corrected calcium | 2.2–2.6 mmol/L |
| serum phosphate | 0.8–1.4 mmol/L |
| serum total protein | 61–76 g/L |
| serum albumin | 37–49 g/L |
| serum total bilirubin | 1–22 μmol/L |
| serum conjugated bilirubin | 0–3.4 μmol/L |
| serum alanine aminotransferase | 5–35 U/L |
| serum aspartate aminotransferase | 1–31 U/L |
| serum alkaline phosphatase | 45–105 U/L (over 14 years) |
| serum gamma glutamyl transferase | 4–35 U/L (< 50 U/L in males) |
| serum lactate dehydrogenase | 10–250 U/L |
| serum creatine kinase (Males) | 24–195 U/L |
| serum creatine kinase (Females) | 24–170 U/L |
| serum copper | 12–26 μmol/L |
| serum caeruloplasmin | 200–350 mg/L |
| serum urate (males) | 0.23–0.46 mmol/L |
| serum urate (females) | 0.19–0.36 mmol/L |
| plasma lactate | 0.6–1.8 mmol/L |
| plasma ammonia | 12–55 μmol/L |
| fasting plasma glucose | 3.0–6.0 mmol/L |
| haemoglobin A1c (HbA1c) | 3.8–6.4% |
| serum amylase | 60–180 U/L |
| **Blood gases (breathing air at sea level)** | |
| blood $H^+$ | 35–45 nmol/L |
| pH | 7.36–7.44 |
| $paO_2$ | 11.3–12.6 kPa |

| | |
|---|---|
| $PaCO_2$ | 4.7–6.0 kPa |
| base excess | ± 2 mmol/L |
| carboxyhaemoglobin: | |
| non-smoker | < 2% |
| smoker | 3–15% |

**Tumour markers**

| | |
|---|---|
| serum alpha-fetoprotein | < 10 kU/L |
| serum human chorionic gonadotrophin | < 5 U/L |
| serum prostate-specific antigen | males under 40 <2 μg/L<br>males over 40 <4 μg/L |

**Urine**

| | |
|---|---|
| total protein | < 0.2g/24h |
| serum albumin | < 30 mg/24 h |
| calcium | 2.5–7.5 mmol/24h |
| 5-hydroxyindoleacetic acid | 10–47 μmol/24h |

**Immunology/rheumatology**

| | |
|---|---|
| serum C-reactive protein | < 10 mg/L |

# CHAPTER 1

# Cardiology

The aim of this section is to consider the clinical features and management of the common cardiac conditions encountered in hospitals by the general physician, including the management of pericarditis, tamponade, endocarditis, the acute coronary syndromes, cardiac failure, atrial fibrillation, and pacemakers. Questions in the exam may also tackle the common invasive and non-invasive investigations, and the clinical relevance of their results. Note that, whereas you may be required to make difficult diagnoses from simple investigations (e.g. ECGs), you may also be required to make simple diagnoses from difficult investigations (e.g. transthoracic echocardiograms).

## NORMAL VALUES

| | |
|---|---|
| creatine kinase MB fraction | < 5% |
| serum troponin I | 0–0.4 μg/L |
| serum troponin T | 0–0.1 μg/L |

# Questions

## Question 1

A 46-year-old man presents six weeks after an anterior myocardial infarction with occasional new symptoms of angina that are unresponsive to medical treatment, and dyspnoea. The ECG demonstrates persistent elevation of ST segments. He reports that he has felt palpitations on several occasions in the preceding few weeks. A 24-hour tape records recurrent trains of ventricular tachycardia. On examination, the jugular venous pressure is not raised. Cardiac auscultation reveals a displaced apex beat +1 cm laterally, normal heart sounds with no murmurs. The most likely diagnosis is:

A a further anterior myocardial infarction

B left ventricular aneurysm

C Dressler's syndrome

D pericarditis

E ventricular septal defect

## Question 2

A 44-year-old man presents with a week's history of fever (38.8°C on admission). On further enquiry, he reports an approximately two-week history of fatigue, weakness and night sweats. On examination, he has conjunctival petechiae and a systolic flow murmur. Three sets of blood cultures demonstrate *S. bovis* infection. He is successfully treated for infective endocarditis. Transthoracic and transoesophageal echocardiograms had both demonstrated vegetations. Which of the following investigations would be most appropriate to organise prior to discharge?

A erythrocyte sedimentation rate

B anti-nuclear antibody

C transoesophageal echocardiography

D colonoscopy

E no further investigations are necessary

## Question 3

A previously well 28-year-old woman presents with a history of transient ischaemic attacks affecting her right side and her speech. She had returned to the United Kingdom after a holiday to Australia, two days previously. She noted that one of her thighs had been swollen, hot and tender to touch. There was nothing to find in her blood investigations including routine haematology and biochemistry, ECG, chest x-ray, and CT brain. The most likely diagnosis is:

A atrial myxoma

B carotid artery stenosis

C embolism from paroxysmal atrial fibrillation

D patent foramen ovale

E subarachnoid haemorrhage

## Question 4

A 63-year-old retired male presented with a three-week history of progressive dyspnoea and swollen ankles. Further history was not reliable, as he appeared to be confused. He confessed to smoking 30 cigarettes per day, but was vague about his alcohol intake. He had been living on sandwiches for the previous year. On examination, he was drowsy and confused, with an MTS of 8 out of 10. The heart rate was 130/minute, and the blood pressure measured 110/74 mmHg. The JVP was not raised. On examination, the apex was displaced to the anterior axillary line and, on auscultation, there was an added third heart sound. Auscultation of the lung fields revealed fine inspiratory crackles. On abdominal examination, there was palpable hepatomegaly 6 cm below the costal margin. Both ankles were swollen. Neurological examination revealed mild weakness in both lower limbs and absent ankle and knee jerks. The sensation was normal. Investigations were as follows: ECG – sinus tachycardia, with large QRS voltages; chest film – enlarged cardiothoracic ratio and bilateral pleural effusions

| **Blood tests:** | |
|---|---|
| haemoglobin | 9 g/dL |
| white cell count | 6 × $10^9$/L |
| platelet count | 90 × $10^9$/L |
| MCV | 103 fL |
| serum sodium | 131 mmol/L |
| serum potassium | 5 mmol/L |
| serum urea | 11 mmol/L |
| serum creatinine | 90 μmol/L |
| splerum bicarbonate | 11 mmol/L |
| plasma glucose | 6 mmol/L |
| **Arterial gases, on air:** | |
| pH | 7.23 |
| $pCO_2$ | 3.4 kPa |
| $pO_2$ | 9.2 kPa |
| **ECG:** | sinus tachycardia, with large QRS voltages |
| **Chest film:** | enlarged cardiothoracic and bilateral pleural effusions |

What is the most probable unifying diagnosis?

A alcoholic cardiomyopathy

B thiamine deficiency

C infective endocarditis

D polyarteritis nodosa

E congestive cardiac failure

## Question 5

A 69-year-old man presented for a routine cardiology appointment. He had been discharged three weeks previously, having sustained a first myocardial infarction. An echocardiogram performed one week previously had demonstrated left ventricular dysfunction. Examination revealed a regular pulse of 106 beats per minute, a blood pressure of 115/72, and no evidence of cardiac failure. Renal function was slightly abnormal. His medication included ramipril 10 mg per day and aspirin 75 mg daily. What would be the most appropriate medication to add to his current therapeutic regimen?

A amlodipine

B bendroflumethiazide (bendrofluazide)

C carvedilol

D digoxin

E isosorbide mononitrate

## Question 6

An 18-year-old man presents with a history of dizziness on standing, which has developed over the last month. The most recent episode occurred while he was shopping; his mother says that he suddenly became hot, dizzy, and fell to the floor shaking. He appeared to be unconscious for only a few seconds. There was no history of incontinence or tongue biting. He recovered very quickly, with no evidence of confusion or disorientation. What is the likely diagnosis?

A complex partial seizures

B generalised tonic-clonic seizures

C pseudoseizures

D syncope

E cataplexy

## Question 7

A 60-year-old female was being seen by her GP with hypertension and congestive cardiac failure. She was prescribed a combination of frusemide 120 mg and enalapril 5 mg once daily. She was normotensive on this combination and had no symptoms of heart failure. Blood tests performed at the time of commencing the medications revealed a serum urea of 18 mmol/L and a serum creatinine of 300 µmol/L. Four months after commencing therapy, she presented with nausea, malaise and pallor. Blood pressure was 160/100 mmHg. The patient was not fluid-overloaded.

**Blood tests:**

| | |
|---|---|
| haemoglobin | 9 g/L |
| white cell count | $5 \times 10^9$/L |
| MCV | 88 fL |
| serum sodium | 134 mmol/L |
| serum potassium | 5.6 mmol/L |
| serum urea | 36 mmol/L |
| serum creatinine | 600 µmol/L |

What will be the best initial management step?

A decrease the dose of enalapril

B decrease the dose of frusemide

C stop the enalapril

D stop the frusemide

E stop both drugs

## Question 8

At presentation of a chest pain, the ECG of a 37-year-old man demonstrates the development of a tall, initial R wave, ST depression and tall, upright T waves in V1 and V2. The most likely diagnosis is an acute myocardial infarction in a territory that is best described as:

A anterior

B anteroseptal

C anterolateral

D inferior

E posterior

## Question 9

A 30-year-old plumber presented with a four-hour history of sudden onset of severe left flank pain. He had no past medical history. He was divorced three years ago. He had consumed 7–10 units of alcohol per day, and smoked 20–30 cigarettes per day. On examination, he was distressed with pain. The temperature was 37.8°C. The heart rate was 120 beats per minute, and irregularly irregular. The blood pressure was 80/40 mmHg. On auscultation, there was a soft systolic murmur in the mitral area and an added third heart sound. The chest was clear. Abdominal examination revealed marked tenderness in the left flank. Investigations were as follows:

| **Blood tests:** | |
|---|---|
| haemoglobin | 12 g/L |
| white cell count | $11 \times 10^9$/L |
| platelet count | $98 \times 10^9$/L |
| MCV | 105 fL |
| serum urea and electrolytes | normal |
| **ECG:** | atrial fibrillation; tall R waves and T wave inversion in the lateral leads |
| **CXR:** | cardiomegaly |
| **Urinalysis:** | blood (+), protein (+), no growth |

What was the most probable cause of the flank pain?

A splenic rupture

B acute pancreatitis

C perforated peptic ulcer

D mesenteric infarction

E left renal infarction

## Question 10

A 50-year-old man presents to Casualty with chest pain, having been previously fit and well. His electrocardiogram on admission shows an inferior myocardial infarction. The patient had been treated by the London Ambulance Service simply through thrombolysis, but he is supposed to be fast-tracked for PTCA. He develops complete heart block, which is accompanied by hypotension with a blood pressure of 90/60 mmHg. A temporary pacing wire is inserted and his blood pressure returns to 110/75 mmHg. Four hours after insertion of the pacing wire he becomes cold and clammy and his blood pressure falls to 70/40 mmHg. His electrocardiogram shows a paced rhythm of 70 beats per minute. What is the most likely diagnosis?

**A** aortic dissection

**B** lead displacement

**C** pacing wire perforation causing ventricular rupture

**D** reinfarction

**E** ruptured chordae resulting in severe regurgitation

## Question 11

A 56-year-old man, with long standing rheumatoid arthritis of more than 20 years, presents with signs of fluid retention: raised jugular venous pressure +5 cm, bibasal crepitations, pitting leg oedema bilaterally, and tender hepatomegaly +3 cm below costal margin. Echocardiogram is suggestive of a cardiomyopathy, and examination is otherwise normal apart from a laterally displaced apex beat +1 cm, and macroglossia. He has been taking methotrexate and NSAIDs for his rheumatoid disease; his previous medication history is unremarkable apart from penicillamine, which around 12 years ago he had taken for a year, before discontinuation as a result of adverse effects. The best investigation to secure the diagnosis is:

**A** gallium scan

**B** 24-hour Holter ECG monitoring

**C** 12-lead ECG

**D** rectal biopsy

**E** autoimmune screen

## Question 12

A 65-year-old man presents with severe central crushing chest pain. ECG demonstrates evidence of an inferior myocardial infarction. He receives TPA, heparin and aspirin. Four hours after presentation, he starts to feel dizzy and breathless, his pulse is 40 bpm regular, blood pressure is 80/50, heart sounds are soft, and chest is clear to auscultation. ECG demonstrates 2:1 block with T wave inversion inferiorly. Intravenous atropine is administered, to no effect. The next best management step is:

A i.v. dopamine

B i.v. isoprenaline

C insertion of a permanent pacemaker

D insertion of a temporary pacing wire

E monitor conservatively

## Question 13

A 29-year-old man presents to hospital with a six-hour history of palpitations and breathlessness at rest. His echocardiogram on admission demonstrates atrial fibrillation with a ventricular rate of 140 beats per minute. His blood pressure is 130/60. What is the best pharmacological agent for cardioversion?

A intravenous digoxin

B intravenous esmolol

C oral verapamil

D oral sotalol

E oral flecainide

## Question 14

Which of the following conditions is a recognised indication for permanent pacing?

A arrhythmogenic right ventricular dysplasia

B nocturnal Wenckebach

C PR interval > 300 milliseconds

D asymptomatic bifascicular block

E hypertrophic obstructive cardiomyopathy

## Questions 15 and 16

A 22-year-old man presents with collapse without warning. His echocardiogram is normal, but the resting ECG is abnormal. Two siblings have died of unexplained causes. He is deaf, as were his deceased siblings.

## Question 15

What is the most likely molecular diagnosis?

A abnormal potassium channel

B abnormal sodium channel

C abnormal calcium channel

D abnormal chloride channel

E abnormal magnesium channel

## Question 16

What would be the best initial treatment for his cardiological condition?

A atenolol

B do nothing

C flecainide

D digoxin

E verapamil

## Question 17

A 72-year-old man is noted to have a systolic murmur and undergoes a transthoracic echocardiogram, which demonstrates aortic stenosis. Which of the following is associated with a poor prognosis in this patient?

A clinical features of left ventricular failure

B cardiomegaly on chest x-ray

C aortic root dilatation

D severe valvular calcification on echocardiogram

E left ventricular hypertrophy on ECG criteria

## Question 18

A 50-year-old gentleman with known severe aortic stenosis develops syncopal symptoms on exertion. He was known to have hypertension and hypercholesterolaemia, and a coronary angiogram had been performed to assess for coronary artery disease (and was unremarkable). What is the next step in his management?

A aortic valvuloplasty

B aortic valve replacement

C close outpatient follow-up with serial echocardiograms

D exercise testing with identification of arrhythmia

E observe until symptoms disappear

## Question 19

A 15-year-old boy with breathlessness and cyanosis is subject to a cardiac catheter investigation. The data were as follows:

| *Chamber* | *Pressure (mmHg)* | *Oxygen saturation (%)* |
|---|---|---|
| SVC | | 46 |
| IVC | | 43 |
| RA | 8 | 45 |
| RV | 104/12 | 45 |
| PA | 23/8 | 44 |
| LV | 90/3 | 83 |
| Ao | 100/55 | 60 |

What is the diagnosis?

A VSD with a left-to-right shunt

B VSD with a right-to-left shunt

C patent ductus arteriosus with a left-to-right shunt

D VSD with a right-to-left shunt and severe pulmonary stenosis

E Fallot's tetralogy

# Answers to Chapter 1: Cardiology

These solutions aim to provide the reason(s) for the right answer, and also the reason(s) for the wrong answers being excluded.

1 **Answer B:** This is a typical history of a left ventricular aneurysm. The patient having presented with anterior myocardial infarction originally, option A is less likely, and there are no other features in the history to support this. Dressler's syndrome usually presents 1–4 weeks following an infarct, and is a syndrome that consists of recurrent pericarditis, pleural effusions, fever, anaemia and a high erythrocyte sedimentation rate. Pericarditis normally occurs acutely (i.e. within the first few days) and transiently, but may occur with anterior or inferior infarcts. A ventricular septal defect, in this context, would be associated with high venous pressures, and a murmur at the left sternal edge should be audible.

2 **Answer D:** The non-specific symptoms reported by this man are most likely due to infective endocarditis, rather than another cause (such as systemic lupus erythematosus, alluded to in the option B). The portal of entry of *S. bovis* bacteraemia is the GI tract. In rare instances, the urinary tract, the hepatobiliary tree, or the oropharynx have been suspected as the source of the bacteraemia. A strong association exists between *S. bovis* bacteraemia with or without endocarditis and underlying malignancy or premalignant lesions of the colon. It is advised that every patient with *S. bovis* bacteraemia with or without endocarditis should be examined for a GI malignancy.

3 **Answer D:** This is a case of stroke in a young person due to prolonged immobility. A deep vein thrombosis ('DVT') with patent foramen ovale ('PFO') would cause paradoxical embolism and stroke. The role of a patent foramen ovale in the aetiology of cerebrovascular events is considered controversial. Around 15% of the population have a PFO and these are therefore frequently identified in patients undergoing extensive investigation for unexplained cerebral events. The theoretical mechanism for strokes in such people is passage of a thrombus from the right to the left atrium (paradoxical embolism), and the presence of a DVT in a patient with an otherwise unexplained cerebral event should make one suspicious that a PFO is responsible.

4 **Answer B:** This patient with alcohol dependence syndrome (low platelet count, raised MCV), heart failure, peripheral neuropathy and a severe metabolic acidosis has 'wet beri-beri'. Thiamine deficiency is more common in alcoholics, due to primary dietary deficiency. Thiamine is a co-factor for the enzyme pyruvate dehydrogenase, a vital enzyme for aerobic glycolysis. Insufficient activity of pyruvate DH results in predominantly anaerobic glycolysis and lactic acidosis. Treatment is with thiamine.

5 **Answer C:** Trials have demonstrated that people within 3–21 days of an acute myocardial infarction, on an angiotensin-converting enzyme inhibitor, benefited from carvedilol compared with placebo in terms of mortality and non-fatal acute myocardial infarction (*see* for example the CAPRICORN trial, *Lancet.* 2001; **357**: 1385–90).

6 **Answer D:** The history is typical of syncope, with dizziness on standing, short duration of loss of consciousness, and a quick recovery. A few convulsions may be seen (convulsive syncope), but not tongue biting. The distinction between real generalised seizures and pseudoseizures is often difficult to make, especially in patients who have both. The most helpful clinical features pointing to pseudoseizures are any evidence of voluntary activity during the actual episode (e.g. resistance to eye opening and passive limb movements, gaze aversion, presentation of the patient's own hand falling on face), and absence of papillary dilatation which is said to be invariable in generalised seizures. Complex movements such as flailing of the limbs, rolling of the body or pelvic thrusting are rare in generalised seizures.

As a rough guide, loss of consciousness can be characterised between fits, pseudofits and faints according to these criteria:

| | Fit | Pseudofit | Faint |
|---|---|---|---|
| Age | any age | commonly young female | uncommon in young males |
| Duration | none or short | may be long | may be adequate to avoid a fall |
| Location | anywhere, could be in a dangerous location | always in company | bad locations avoided |
| In sleep | may occur | never | never |
| Provocation | sleep deprivation | lack of attention | hunger and fatigue |

7 **Answer E:** The answer is to stop both drugs. An ACE inhibitor should not be started, certainly if the serum creatinine is at least 300 μmol/L.

8 **Answer E:** The ECG changes described are typical of a posterior infarct.

9 **Answer E:** The differential of a murmur plus fever should raise the possibility of endocarditis, but there is no previous history of being unwell. He clearly has poor LV function (very low BP, third heart sound). The murmur of MR is functional. The atrial fibrillation has predisposed him to an intra-cardiac thrombus, which has embolised to the kidney. However, D is still possible.

10 **Answer C:** The likeliest diagnosis is pacing-wire-induced rupture. The time course in this situation is vital as this often occurs through an infarcted RV wall, which is more friable and thin walled, regardless of the infarct setting.

Reinfarction is unlikely as no mention has been made that the patient has reperfused in the first instance. Ruptured chordae is less likely to happen with an inferior MI than an anterior or lateral MI. Aortic dissection is unlikely given the presentation.

**11 Answer D:** A rectal biopsy should hopefully confirm the diagnosis of amyloidosis. The other options would not specifically secure this diagnosis. The main types of amyloid are AL amyloid (primary amyloidosis), whose signs include oedema, macroglossia, hepatosplenomegaly, carpal tunnel syndrome, and malabsorption; and AA amyloid (secondary amyloidosis), which occurs in chronic infections, inflammation and neoplasma, tending to affect kidneys, liver and spleen, and commonly presenting as proteinuria, nephrosis, and hepatosplenomegaly. Diagnosis is made after Congo Red staining of affected tissue, and the rectum is a favoured site for biopsy (positive in around 80%).

**12 Answer D:** This patient has had an inferior MI, which is commonly associated with conduction abnormalities. He now develops heart block, which leaves him bradycardic, symptomatic, with a low BP. Isoprenaline is contraindicated in acute MI due to its positive ionotropic effects and arrythmogenic potential. A temporary pacing wire would deal with the situation until the inferior MI has fully resolved.

**13 Answer E:** Haemodynamically stable patients with AF can be converted to sinus rhythm through class IC agents such as flecainide. These have the advantage of acting rapidly to convert recent-onset atrial fibrillation to sinus rhythm.

**14 Answer E:** Dual chamber pacing in HOCM may reduce the LV outflow gradient by reversing septal depolarisation, thereby improving cardiac performance. Asymptomatic bifascicular block and PR interval > 300 milliseconds are relatively benign phenomena that require surveillance only. Nocturnal Wenckebach is a normal phenomenon due to high vagal tone and requires no action. Arrythmogenic right ventricular dysplasia is a condition where there is fatty infiltration of right ventricular myocardium, which predisposes to sudden arrhythmic death and often requires aggressive antiarrhythmic therapy or an implantable defibrillator.

**15, 16 Answers A, A:** It is not completely impossible that there may be an applied clinical science question in the Part 2 Examination, even though this is more the domain of Part 1. Deafness and sudden death suggest Jervell-Lange-Nielsen syndrome, which is due to an abnormal potassium channel in the heart and cochlea. ECG demonstrates characteristically QT prolongation, which predisposes to sudden death due to torsades de pointes/VF. It is autosomally recessively inherited. Patients with congenital long QT syndrome presenting with symptoms of syncope are treated with high-dose beta-blockade. (*See* **Learning point.**)

17 **Answer A:** Aortic stenosis has a worse prognosis when accompanied by left ventricular dysfunction. Other poor prognostic factors include increased gradient across the valve (70 mmHg or more), age and symptomatology.

18 **Answer B:** Exertional syncope is an indication for surgery in patients with severe aortic stenosis, even in the absence of exertional dyspnoea. Aortic valvuloplasty compares unfavourably with aortic valve replacement in the medium and long term in aortic stenosis.

19 **Answer E:** The cardiac catheter data demonstrate high right ventricular pressure, a pressure gradient of 57 across the pulmonary artery, low oxygen saturations in all chambers, a right-to-left shunt at ventricular level, and a discrepancy in oxygen saturation between the left ventricle and the aorta. The diagnosis is Fallot's tetralogy. The answer is not D, due to the low saturations in the aorta (meaning that the aorta is overriding the right ventricle).

# Learning Points

### *Questions 15 and 16*

## Learning point

**Causes of a long QT syndrome**

| | |
|---|---|
| Inherited long QT | Jervell-Lange Nielsen syndrome<br>Romano-Ward syndrome |
| Electrolytes | hypokalaemia, hypomagnesaemia, hypocalcaemia |
| Endocrine disorders | hypothyroidism, hyperparathyroidism, phaeochromocytoma |
| Cardiac conditions | myocardial ischaemia, myocardial infarction, myocarditis, bradyarrhythmia, AV nodal block |
| Intracranial disorders | subarachnoid haemorrhage, head trauma, encephalitis |
| Nutritional disorders | anorexia nervosa, starvation |
| Drugs | antiarrhythmics, terfanidine, cisapride, erythromycin,<br>larithromycin, trimethoprim, ketoconazole, itraconazole,<br>haloperidol, pheniothiazines, tricyclic antidepressants |

## CHAPTER 2

# Haematology, oncology and immunology

Clinical haematology in MRCP(UK) has some favourite topics, including iron metabolism, the anaemias, polycythaemia and myeloproliferative disorders, white cell disorders, and disorders of haemostasis. A few questions will be set on immunology, particularly immunological tests, and particularly anaphylaxis, angio-oedema, and urticaria. It is difficult to predict the topics of the oncology section.

## NORMAL VALUES

### Coagulation factors

| | |
|---|---|
| prothrombin time | 11.5–15.5 s |
| international normalised ratio (INR) | < 1.4 |
| activated partial thromboplastin time | 30–40 s |
| fibrinogen | 1.8–5.4 g/L |
| bleeding time | 3–8 m |
| factors II, V, VII, VIII, IX, X, XI, XII | 50–150 IU/dL |
| von Willebrand factor | 45–150 IU/dL |
| von Willebrand factor antigen | 50–150 IU/dL |
| protein C | 80–135 IU/dL |
| protein S | 80–120 IU/dL |
| antithrombin III | 80–120 IU/dL |
| activated protein C resistance | 2.12–4.0 |
| fibrin degradation products | < 100 mg/L |

| | |
|---|---|
| D-Dimer screen | < 0.5 mg/L |
| **Haematinics** | |
| serum iron | 12–30 µmol/L |
| serum iron-binding capacity | 45–75 µmol/L |
| serum ferritin | 15–300 µg/L |
| serum transferrin | 2.0–4.0 g/L |
| serum $B_{12}$ | 160–760 ng/L |
| serum folate | 2.0–11.0µg/L |
| red cell folate | 160–640 µg/L |
| serum haptoglobin | 0.13–1.63 g/L |
| haemoglobin electrophoresis: | |
| haemoglobin A | > 95% |
| haemoglobin $A_2$ | 2–3% |
| haemoglobin F | < 2% |
| **Immunology/Rheumatology** | |
| complement C3 | 65–190 mg/dL |
| complement C4 | 15–50 mg/dL |
| serum immunoglobins: | |
| IgG | 6.0–13.0 g/L |
| IgA | 0.8–3.0 g/L |
| IgM | 0.4–2.5 g/L |
| IgE | < 120 kIU/L |
| serum β2–microglobulin | < 3 mg/L |
| autoantibodies (all serum): | |
| adrenal | Negative at 1:10 Dil. |
| anticentromere antibodies | Negative at 1:40 Dil. |
| anticardiolipin antibody: | |
| IgG | 0–23 |
| IgM | 0–11 |
| anti-double-stranded DNA (ELISA) | 0–73 U/mL |
| antineutrophil cytoplasmic antibodies: | |
| anti-proteinase 3 | Negative |
| anti-MPO | Negative |
| antinuclear antibodies | Negative at 1:20 Dil. |
| ENA | Negative |
| anti Jo-1 | Negative |
| anti La | Negative |
| anti-mitochondrial | Negative at 1:20 Dil. |
| anti-RNP | Negative |

| | |
|---|---|
| anti-Scl-70 | Negative |
| anti-Ro | Negative |
| Sm | Negative |
| anti-smooth muscle | Negative at 1:20 Dil. |
| thyroid colloid and microcosmal antigens | Negative at 1:10 Dil. |
| rheumatoid factor | < 30 kIU/L |

# Questions

## Question 1

A 32-year-old Nigerian lady with sickle cell anaemia (Hb SS) has a history of recurrent back pain. She presents to Casualty with fever and a worsening of the back pain. There is no history of weight loss or night sweats.

**Investigations reveal:**

| | |
|---|---|
| haematology | 5.8 g/L |
| white cell count | $10.2 \times 10^9$/L |
| platelet count | 12% |
| serum total bilirubin | 88 µmol/L |
| absolute reticulocyte % | Normal |

What is the most likely diagnosis?

A aplastic crisis

B drug-induced haemolytic crisis

C malaria

D tuberculosis

E vasoocclusive event

## Question 2

A 19-year-old university student presents to the Accident and Emergency Department with a seven-day history of fever, sore throat and malaise. She has not managed to eat food for several days, particularly because of pharyngitis as well as a loss of appetite. She started menstruating a day previously. On examination, she is icteric.

**Investigations reveal:**

| | |
|---|---|
| haemoglobin | 14 g/L |
| MCV | 89 fL |
| white cell count | $6.5 \times 10^9$/L |
| platelet count | $350 \times 10^9$/L |
| absolute reticulocytes | 0.8% |
| serum total bilirubin | 60 mmol/L |
| serum conjugated bilirubin | 10 mmol/L |
| serum aspartate transaminase | 19 U/L |
| serum alkaline phosphatase | 117 U/L |
| serum albumin | 42 g/L |

What is the most likely diagnosis?

A chronic active autoimmune hepatitis

B toxic shock syndrome

C Gilbert's syndrome

D primary biliary cirrhosis

E auto-immune haemolytic anaemia

## Question 3

A 35-year-old woman, who is known to be 27 weeks pregnant, is admitted with severe headache and blurred vision. She reported no neck stiffness or photophobia. She had no previous medical history; this was her first pregnancy and up until now she had had no complications of pregnancy. She was not on any medication. On clinical examination, the fundal height was +28cm above the symphisis pubis, she had a temperature of 38.1°C, pulse 100 regular, and blood pressure 100/68. Chest and heart sounds were normal. Abdomen was generally non-tender distended, consistent with pregnancy. There was no focal neurological deficit and plantar responses were flexor. She had widespread purpuric lesions on her back and lower limbs. There was no evidence of peripheral oedema.

**Blood tests:**

| | |
|---|---|
| haemoglobin | 8.0 g/L |
| MCV | 106.2 fL |
| white cell count | 24.5 × $10^9$/L |
| platelet count | 35 × $10^9$/L |
| reticulocytes | 13% |
| serum sodium | 140 mmol/L |
| serum potassium | 4.3 mmol/L |
| serum urea | 35.9 mmol/L |
| serum creatinine | 310 μmol/L |
| serum protein | 68 g/L |
| serum albumin | 36 g/L |
| serum total bilirubin | 34 mmol/L |
| serum alanine aminotransferase | 28 U/L |
| serum gamma glutamyl transferase | 50 U/L |
| serum alkaline phosphatase | 100 U/L |
| international normalised ratio | 1.0 |

**Further tests:**

| | |
|---|---|
| **Blood film:** | red cell fragments present |
| **Chest film:** | normal |
| **Urinalysis:** | normal |

The most likely diagnosis is:

A disseminated intravascular coagulopathy

B fatty liver of pregnancy

C HELLP syndrome

D thrombotic thrombocytopaenic purpura

E toxic shock syndrome

## Question 4

A 42-year-old woman was admitted with ascites, which had been increasing over the past two months. She also complained of progressive lethargy and that her skin bruised easily. Her urine was dark but stools were normal coloured. Her previous medical history included a left leg DVT two years ago, and a right calf DVT six months ago. On examination, she appeared pale. She did not drink alcohol, had no previous medical history, and was on no medication apart from warfarin 4 mg od. She was apyrexial and there was no lymphadenopathy. Her pulse was 94, regular, and blood pressure 110/76. Her abdomen was distended with generalised tenderness, and there was + 3 cm hepatomegaly.

**Blood tests:**

| | |
|---|---|
| haemoglobin | 8.9 mmol/L |
| MCV | 76 fL |
| white cell count | $2.9 \times 10^9$/L |
| platelet count | $110 \times 10^9$/L |
| serum sodium | 140 mmol/L |
| serum potassium | 4.3 mmol/L |
| serum urea | 5.9 mmol/L |
| serum creatinine | 93 µmol/L |
| serum total protein | 68 g/L |
| serum albumin | 33 g/L |
| serum total bilirubin | 19 mmol/L |
| serum alanine transferase | 68 U/L |
| serum alkaline phosphatase | 110 U/L |
| international normalised ratio | 1.0 |

**Further tests:**

| | |
|---|---|
| **Urinalysis:** | evidence of haemosiderin |
| **Ultrasound of the abdomen:** | hepatomegaly with enlarged caudate lobe<br>no blood flow in the hepatic veins<br>gross ascites<br>bowel gas overlying pancreas; view obscured |

The patient also demonstrated an iron-deficiency anaemia, attributed by her GP to heavy periods. She had been on iron supplements consequently.

The most helpful test to establish the underlying diagnosis is:

**A** bone marrow aspirate and trephine

**B** haemoglobin electrophoresis

**C** Ham's test

**D** osmotic fragility studies

**E** serum homocysteine levels

## Question 5

A 71-year-old retired journalist is admitted to the Casualty department with back pain, having fallen in his garden and sustained a fractured neck of femur. The orthopaedic surgeons wish to operate on him but they note his abnormal blood results on admission and ask the medical team to review him. He has lost about 9 kg in weight and his appetite is poor. He has complained of worsening pain over his lower back and ribs. He has also told his wife that he feels increasingly lethargic. On examination, he looks cachectic. His left leg is shortened, and externally rotated. He is tender to palpation over his T10 vertebra. His pulse is 72/minute regular, and blood pressure 178/84. Physical examination is otherwise normal.

**Blood tests:**

| | |
|---|---|
| haemoglobin | 6.8 g/dL |
| MCV | 88 fL |
| white cell count | $6.2 \times 10^9$/L |
| platelet count | $130 \times 10^9$/L |
| erythrocyte sedimentation rate | 96 mm/hr (Westergren) |
| serum sodium | 135 mmol/L |
| serum potassium | 4.7 mmol/L |
| serum urea | 18.3 mmol/L |
| serum creatinine | 294 µmol/L |
| serum corrected calcium | 2.96 mmol/L |
| serum phosphate | 1.3 mmol/L |
| serum total protein | 85 g/L |
| serum albumin | 38 g/L |
| serum total bilirubin | 12 µmol/L |
| serum alanine transferase | 18 U/L |
| serum alkaline phosphatase | 50 U/L |

**Further tests:**

| | |
|---|---|
| **Blood film:** | marked rouleaux formation |
| **Urinalysis:** | protein (++); blood (++) |
| **X-ray scan of spine:** | changes consistent with osteoporosis |

The most likely diagnosis is:

A chronic myeloid leukaemia

B monoclonal gammopathy of undetermined significance (MGUS)

C myeloma

D myelofibrosis

E Waldenstrom's macroglobulinaemia

## Question 6

A 60-year-old man presented with sudden loss of vision in the left eye. Over the past three months he had noticed increased lethargy, nosebleeds on a couple of occasions, and loss of weight. He had no previous medical history. On examination, his temperature was 37.4°C, pulse 90 regular, and blood pressure 146/92. Cardiovascular and respiratory examinations were entirely normal. Abdominal examination revealed palpable splenomegaly. Cranial nerve examination was normal.

| **Blood tests:** | | |
|---|---|---|
| haemoglobin | 8.8 g/L | |
| MCV | 108 fL | |
| white cell count | $8.2 \times 10^9$/L | |
| neutrophils | $5.0 \times 10^9$/L | |
| lymphocytes | $3.0 \times 10^9$/L | |
| monocytes | $0.2 \times 10^9$/L | |
| platelet count | $430 \times 10^9$/L | |
| erythrocyte sedimentation rate | 150 mm/hr (Westergren) | |
| serum total protein | 90 g/L | |
| serum albumin | 36 g/L | |
| immunoglobulins | IgG | 1.9 |
| | IgA | 1.2 |
| | IgM | 40.3 |

**Radiology:** skeletal survey – reported as normal.

The most likely diagnosis is:

A chronic myeloid leukaemia

B monoclonal gammopathy of undetermined significance (MGUS)

C myeloma

D myelofibrosis

E Waldenstrom's macroglobulinaemia

## Question 7

A 13-year-old boy was referred because of recurrent bouts of abdominal pain and tiredness to his GP, who referred him to the Metabolic Clinic. This was the fourth time it had happened but previously these attacks had resolved spontaneously. Three days ago, he had developed a sore throat, myalgia and headache. He had no previous medical history, and was not on any medication. There had been, however, a family history of abdominal discomfort. On examination, he was mildly jaundiced. His temperature was 37.3°C, pulse 98 regular and blood pressure 100/65. Cardiovascular and respiratory examinations were entirely normal. On palpation of his abdomen, there was +4 cm splenomegaly.

**Blood tests:**

| | |
|---|---|
| haemoglobin | 11.5 g/L |
| MCV | 100.3 fL |
| white cell count | $4.2 \times 10^9$/L |
| platelet count | $160 \times 10^9$/L |
| total protein | 70 g/L |
| serum albumin | 42 g/L |
| serum total bilirubin | 44 mmol/L |
| serum alanine aminotransferase | 25 U/L |
| serum alkaline phosphatase | 125 U/L |
| serum gamma glutamyl transferase | 35 U/L |

**Further tests:**

| | |
|---|---|
| **Direct Coombs' test:** | negative |
| **Urinalysis:** | urobilinogen (++), no bilirubin |

A blood film had previously demonstrated spherocytes.

The most helpful test to confirm the diagnosis is:

A bone marrow aspirate and trephine

B haemoglobin electrophoresis

C Ham's test

D osmotic fragility studies

E Schumm's test

## Question 8

A 19-year-old man awaiting an elective hernia repair was referred to the ENT Registrar on call because of a severe nosebleed. He had suffered greatly with nosebleeds in the past; he had also tended to bruise easily. He was adopted and knew nothing of his real parents. He was at the time of presentation on no medication. In searching through his medical notes, it was noted that he had been admitted under the maxillo-facial surgeons for extraction of his wisdom teeth. The only concern at the time had been that he required suturing. On examination, he was apyrexial. He had bruises all over his skin, but otherwise there was absolutely nothing else to detect on physical examination. His nose bleed had stopped spontaneously.

**Blood tests:**

| | |
|---|---|
| haemoglobin | 13.5 g/L |
| MCV | 79 |
| APTT | 78 |
| APTT with 50:50 mix of normal plasma | 44 |
| PT | 13 s |
| TT | 20 s |
| bleeding time | 18 m |
| Factor VIII | 11% |
| Factor IX | 65% |

[The full blood count including platelet count had been recorded as normal.]

The most likely diagnosis is:

A antiphospholipid syndrome, associated with systemic lupus erythematosus

B circulating antibody to factor VII

C haemophilia A

D haemophilia B

E von Willebrand disease

## Question 9

A 26-year-old lady of African-Carribean ethnic background presents in acute shock at 35 weeks of pregnancy with profuse vaginal bleeding. She has suffered two previous miscarriages. She has a pulse of 112 beats per minute, blood pressure of 80/64 mmHg and no foetal heart sounds are audible.

**Investigations reveal:**

| | |
|---|---|
| haemoglobin | 9.5 g/L |
| platelet count | $66 \times 10^9$/L |
| prothrombin time | 21 s |
| white cell count | $11 \times 10^9$/L |
| activated partial thromboplastin time | 52 s |
| fibrinogen concentration | 0.5 g/L |

serum urea and electrolytes were normal.

What is the most appropriate next step in the management?

A antithrombin III infusion

B fibrinogen replacement infusion (cryoprecipitate)

C intravenous heparin

D platelet transfusion

E transfusion of two units of group O Rhesus D negative blood

## Question 10

An 84-year-old woman presented to her GP with non-specific tiredness. On examination, she was anaemic but had no palpable splenomegaly. Investigations revealed a haemoglobin of 9.7 g/dL. She was commenced on oral iron therapy for one month and her haemoglobin remained unchanged.

**Further investigations revealed:**

| | |
|---|---|
| MCV | 102 fL |
| serum ferritin | 70 ug/L |
| vitamin $B_{12}$ | 280 ng/L |
| red cell folate | 230 ug/L |
| serum urea | 9.1 mmol/L |
| serum creatinine | 150 µmol/L |

**Blood film:** marked anisopoikilocytosis

What is the most likely diagnosis?

A aplastic anaemia

B anaemia due to renal disease

C hypothyroidism

D iron deficiency anaemia

E sideroblastic anaemia

## Question 11

A 47-year-old man with a known history of peripheral vascular disease, is admitted for an elective left femoral-popliteal bypass operation. Peripheral pulses were present, but weak distally on admission. Blood investigations including full blood count and biochemistry on admission had been normal. He was commenced appropriately on a heparin infusion, and the procedure itself was uneventful. Four days following the procedure, just as the patient was due to go home, he complained of a purpuric rash.

| | |
|---|---|
| haemoglobin | 11.2 g/L |
| white cell count | $12 \times 10^9$/L |
| platelet count | $36 \times 10^9$/L |
| international normalised ratio | 1.2 |
| prothrombin time and activated partial protrombin time (PT and APTT) | normal |

What is the best initial treatment strategy?

**A** take the patient back to theatre to examine graft patency

**B** stop any form of anticoagulation, including heparin infusion

**C** commence warfarin

**D** commence hirudin

**E** give a transfusion of platelets

## Questions 12 and 13

A 12-year-old boy received the first dose of chemotherapy for Hodgkin's lymphoma. Electrolytes taken 48 hours later were as follows:

| | |
|---|---|
| serum sodium | 136 mmol/L |
| serum potassium | 7.1 mmol/L |
| serum urea | 16 mmol/L |
| serum creatinine | 260 µmol/L |
| serum phosphate | 3.9 mmol/L |
| serum urate | 1.0 mmol/L |

## Question 12

How do you best explain the electrolyte abnormalities?

A tumour lysis syndrome

B rhabdomyolysis

C acute tubulointerstitial nephritis secondary to allopurinol

D haemolysed sample

E renal tubular acidosis

## Question 13

What is the cause of the patient's renal failure?

A ureteric obstruction by tumour

B retroperitoneal fibrosis

C renal amyloidosis

D hyperuricaemia nephropathy

E malignant hypercalcaemia

## Question 14

A 35-year-old woman on chemotherapy complained of difficulty in buttoning her clothes, hesitancy in micturition and unsteady gait. She also had colicky abdominal pain. Examination revealed a palpable bladder, and an empty rectum.

Which cytotoxic drug is most likely to have caused her problems?

A cyclophosphamide

B doxorubicin

C fludarabine

D methotrexate

E vincristine

## Question 15

A 57-year-old man is treated for a low grade non-Hodgkin's lymphoma. He then presents with lethargy. Examination reveals a pale man with generalised lymphadenopathy. Abdominal examination reveals a spleen palpable +12 cm below the costal margin. His medication comprises chlorambucil and prednisolone.

| **Investigations reveal:** | |
|---|---|
| haemoglobin | 6.3 g/L |
| MCV | 82 fL |
| white cell count | $2 \times 10^9$/L |
| platelet count | $92 \times 10^9$/L |
| reticulocyte count | 1.8% |
| **Blood film:** | pancytopaenia |

What is the most likely diagnosis?

A marrow suppression by chlorambucil

B hypersplenism

C anaemia of chronic disease

D haemolytic anaemia due to lymphoma

E leukaemic transformation

## Question 16

A 57-year-old man presented with deteriorating breathlessness over the last year. He had received inhalers for the last two years prescribed by his GP, which he had, up until the last three months, used intermittently. He was also taking ramipril 10 mg od and bendroflumethiazine (bendrofluazide) 2.5 mg daily for a six year history of hypertension. He had stopped smoking two years previously and consumed approximately 14 units of alcohol weekly. On examination he was cyanosed and had a swollen face and dilated superficial veins over the anterior chest wall with fixed dilated neck veins. His blood pressure was 154/88 mmHg, pulse was 88 beats per minute. Heart sounds were normal. There was pitting oedema of the ankles. Respiratory examination revealed a hyperexpanded chest with scattered expiratory wheeze. Abdominal examination was normal.

**Investigations revealed:**

**Blood tests:**

| | |
|---|---|
| haemoglobin | 14.8 g/L |
| white cell count | $12.9 \times 10^9$/L |
| platelet count | $488 \times 10^9$/L |
| serum sodium | 130 mmol/L |
| serum urea | 10.8 mmol/L |
| serum corrected calcium | 2.81 mmol/L |

**Further tests:**

| | |
|---|---|
| **ECG:** | normal |
| **Chest x-ray:** | hyperexpanded lung fields with left paratracheal shadowing |
| **CT scan of the thorax:** | anterior mediastinal mass |

Which single investigation would be most helpful in making a diagnosis?

A biopsy of the mediastinal mass

B bone marrow trephine biopsy

C bronchoscopy

D CT scan of the abdomen

E tuberculin skin test

## Question 17

A 57-year-old lady was admitted to hospital with increasing thirst and generalised abdominal pain. She had been diagnosed with breast carcinoma three years previously, and treated with a radical mastectomy.

**Investigations revealed:**

| | |
|---|---|
| serum corrected calcium | 3.5 mmol/L |
| serum alkaline phosphatase | 1110 U/L |

Her serum calcium was still elevated following four litres of 0.9% N saline intravenous infusion. Which of the following is the most appropriate next step?

A 8 mg dexamethasone

B intravenous 0.9% N saline over four hours

C low calcium diet

D intravenous 90 mg pamidronate

E radiotherapy

## Question 18

A 28-year-old man was referred to clinic by his GP. Over the past two months he had noticed increasing exertional dyspnoea. Previously, he had been physically active and jogged regularly. At the time of referral he was breathless climbing one flight of stairs. He has a past history of asthma and underwent an orchidopexy as a child for an undescended right testis. On examination, gynaecomastia was noted. No wheeze was audible in his chest. Examination of the genitals revealed a firm mass 1 cm × 1 cm in the right testis.

**Investigations revealed:**

| | |
|---|---|
| serum alpha-fetoprotein | 90 kU/L |
| serum beta-human chorionic gonadotrophin | 28267 U/L |

What is the most likely diagnosis?

A choriocarcinoma

B gonadoblastoma

C Leydig cell tumour

D seminoma

E Sertoli cell tumour

## Question 19

A 55-year-old man was referred to the Outpatient clinic with anaemia. He had presented to his GP with a three-month history of fatigue and low back pain. There was no preceeding history of trauma. A plain x-ray of his lumbar spine showed a lytic lesion in the body of the fourth lumbar vertebra (L4).

| **Investigations revealed:** | |
|---|---|
| haemoglobin | 10.5 g/L |
| white cell count | $4.0 \times 10^9$/L |
| platelet count | $175 \times 10^9$/L |
| serum sodium | 137 mmol/L |
| serum potassium | 3.5 mmol/L |
| serum urea | 2.7 mmol/L |
| serum creatinine | 110 µmol/L |
| serum corrected calcium | 2.4 mmol/L |

| **Further tests:** | |
|---|---|
| **Urinalysis:** | Bence Jones protein detected |
| **Skeletal survey:** | increased uptake in the L4 region |

Which of the following therapies will reduce the risk of pathological fracture?

A autologous stem cell transplantation

B melphalan

C pamidronate

D plasmapharesis

E steroids

## Question 20

After presenting with an upper gastrointestinal bleed and back pain, a 92-year-old lady was diagnosed with gastric carcinoma. Subsequent investigations revealed multiple bony metastases in the spine and metastases in the liver and lungs. She was discharged home on oramorph for pain relief, but was readmitted within 48 hours because of increased pain. One week after readmission she developed a productive cough, and a chest radiograph demonstrated consolidation at the right base on the chest x-ray. Within a few hours, her condition deteriorated rapidly, and she became drowsy, with laboured breathing. What is now the next best management step for the doctor to discuss with the patient's relatives?

**A** intravenous antibiotics and fentanyl patch

**B** intravenous antibiotics and intravenous fluids

**C** intravenous antibiotics and oramorph

**D** subcutaneous diamorphine as required

**E** subcutaneous diamorphine pump

## Question 21

Vanessa is a 31-year-old female patient who presented at Casualty in respiratory distress and unable to swallow her own saliva. The problem had begun following a routine dental extraction. She was apyrexial and there was no obvious skin rash. She was successfully intubated despite marked pharyngeal and laryngeal oedema, and her chest x-ray film was normal. Following recovery, she admitted to a history of recurrent severe attacks of acute, transient, painless, non-itchy swellings over the last five years. These usually occurred on the limbs and trunk. The swellings came on suddenly, grew over a period of 2½ hours, and lasted for 48 hours.

Which of the following is not true of her condition?

**A** it is associated with deficiency of C1 esterase inhibitor

**B** it is characteristically painful

**C** an acquired form occurs in lymphoproliferative disease

**D** an acquired form occurs in pregnancy

**E** it may be treated with danazol

## Question 22

A 50-year-old man presents with a six week history of general malaise and a two-day history of right foot drop, left ulnar nerve palsy, and a widespread purpuric rash. He complains of arthralgia but has no clinical evidence of inflammatory joint disease. Echocardiogram is normal, blood cultures are negative, erythrocyte sedimentation rate 100 mm/hr, ANCA negative, ANA negative, rheumatoid factor strongly positive, C3 0.8 g/L (NR 0.75–1.6), C4 0.02 g/L (0.14–0.5). Dipstix urinary analysis shows blood (++), but no protein.

What is the most likely diagnosis?

**A** ANA negative SLE

**B** cryoglobulinaemia

**C** infective endocarditis

**D** polyarteritis nodosa

**E** rheumatoid arthritis

## Question 23

A 16-year-old man presents with a history of recurrent bacterial sinus infections, and chronic diarrhoeal infections. His mother has a history of rheumatoid arthritis and coeliac disease, and he has been treated in the past with antibiotics. There is nothing to find on examination apart from mild eczema; in particular, there is no organomegaly, and bloods (excluding immunoglobulins) are normal. Levels of IgG and IgM are normal.

The most likely diagnosis is:

**A** X-linked infantile agammaglobulinaemia

**B** selective IgA deficiency

**C** complement deficiency

**D** common variable immunodeficiency

**E** Wiskott-Aldrich syndrome

## Question 24

A 45-year-old woman was admitted to hospital with difficulty breathing. She was admitted from a local restaurant after becoming suddenly unwell while eating curry. On arrival in Casualty, her face and lips were noted to be grossly swollen and there was an audible inspiratory wheeze. There was no past history of allergies. She had been diagnosed with hypertension by her GP and had started on captopril 10 days previously.

**Investigations revealed:**

| | |
|---|---|
| serum IgE | >1000 kU/L |
| mast cell tryptase | normal (after 30 minutes) |

What is the most likely diagnosis?

A C1 inhibitor deficiency

B captopril-induced angioedema

C hyperimmunoglobulinaemia E

D mastocytosis

E nut allergy

# Answers to Chapter 2: Haematology, oncology and immunology

These solutions aim to provide the reason(s) for the right answer, and also the reason(s) for the wrong answers being excluded.

1 **Answer E:** The blood results are suggestive of a sickling episode. The haemoglobin is slightly lower than one would expect normally, with a raised reticulocyte count and hyperbilirubinaemia. There is no evidence of an aplastic crisis as the Hb is reasonable with a good reticulocyte count. Conversely, the haemoglobin concentration is not low enough, and reticulocyte count and serum total bilirubin not high enough, for a haemolytic crisis. Vasoocclusive events can cause bone pain. Triggers include infection, dehydration, alcohol and change in temperature. Likely infection is the cause in this case, as patient has fever. TB and malaria are not as likely from the clinical scenario. Homozygotes for HbS can get malaria. (*See* **Learning point**.)

2 **Answer C:** The level of unconjugated bilirubin is elevated in the absence of any other liver function test abnormalities. From the history given, it appears that the hyperbilirubinaemia occurred following an upper respiratory tract infection that may have been viral; this illness has been associated with anorexia. When calorie intake falls, the plasma levels of unconjugated bilirubin can double, and this rise may be sufficient to produce clinical jaundice in patients with Gilbert's syndrome, which is also associated with fasting, alcohol and menstruation. A nicotinic acid provocation test can also be used as an alternative.

3 **Answer D:** This patient who is pregnant has features of fever, low platelet count with associated bruising, impaired renal function, neurological changes, and evidence of MAHA (microangiopathic haemolytic anemia): all features of TTP. Note that the combination of bloody diarrhoea, haemolytic anaemia and thrombocytopaenia but normal clotting, would have been indicative of haemolytic-uraemic syndrome – in combination with renal failure. This is associated with *E. coli* O157 most commonly. TTP occurs in both familial or acquired forms. There is a deficiency in a metalloproteinase, which breaks down high molecular weight multimers of VWF. Treatment is with FFP. (*See* **Learning point**.)

4 **Answer C:** This lady has paroxysmal nocturnal haemoglobinuria, which is a red cell abnormality characterised by the presence of a clone of red cells with an abnormal sensitivity to membrane lysis by complement, because these cells are not any longer protected from lysis by the body's own complement. Patients may present with aplastic anaemia, myelodysplastic syndromes and acute myeloid leukaemia, or with evidence of thrombosis akin to the

Budd-Chiari syndrome, deep vein thrombosis, and cerebral vein thrombosis. The degree of the haematological abnormalities may vary. Anaemia may be severe enough to warrant transfusion. Reticulocyte counts vary from < 1% to 40%, and neutrophil and platelet counts also vary widely. The blood film may be unremarkable, and the MCV may be high, reflecting the reticulocytosis. Haptoglobins are usually absent and Hb electrophoresis normal. In Ham's test, complement in the patient's serum is activated by acidification to a pH of 6.5. Acidification activates the alternative complement pathway. The cause is a rare, acquired clonal disorder of marrow stem cells in which there is deficient synthesis of the glycosylphosphatidylinositol anchor, a structure that attaches several surface proteins to the cell membrane, resulting from an X-chromosome gene coding for the PIG-A protein essential for the GPI anchor.

5 **Answer C:** Myeloma is a common cause of pathological fractures in the elderly. Myeloma deposits produce little osteoblastic reaction, so the serum alkaline phosphatase is often normal and a bone scan does not show hot spots of increased uptake. This man has presented with a fracture but his elevated erythrocyte sedimentation rate, hypercalcaemia and renal impairment are suggestive of myeloma. Myeloma is a plasma cell neoplasm occurring mainly in later life, producing increasing quantities of a gamma globulin from the abnormal clone of plasma cells. It can present with vague symptoms of ill-health, bony pains, increased susceptibility to infections, bleeding complications or renal failure. His raised total protein level with normal serum albumin implies the presence of a paraprotein. This patient's anaemia is due to internal blood loss from his hip fracture, marrow infiltration and renal failure. His thrombocytopaenia is due to marrow infiltration. To confirm the correct diagnosis, three investigations should be utilised: (a) serum protein electrophoresis will demonstrate a paraprotein and reduced levels of all immunoglobulin classes (immune paresis); (b) bone marrow (the presence of > 10–15% plasma cells indicates myeloma), and (c) radiological skeletal survey (in patients with myeloma, there may be numerous punched out lesions in the skull, vertebral column, ribs, pelvis and long bones).

6 **Answer E:** This patient presents with lethargy, weight loss, loss of vision, and splenomegaly. The blood results show macrocytic anaemia, lymphocytosis, very raised erythrocyte sedimentation rate and raised IgM. Although there is evidence of immunoparesis, the skeletal survey is normal (i.e. there are no lytic lesions), and therefore myeloma is unlikely. More likely, the diagnosis is Waldenstrom's macroglobulinaemia, a condition which is known to cause a hyperviscosity syndrome (due to the raised IgM), that can result in headaches, cerebrovascular accidents, and thromboses. Bleeding may occur due to paraprotein coating the platelet count. The IgM may present with features of

cryoglobulin: Raynaud's phenomenon, small vessel vasculitis. Renal failure is uncommon.

7 **Answer D:** A teenager presenting with abdominal pain, jaundice, macrocytic anaemia and an increased urinary urobilinogen (Coombs' test/direct antiglobulin test negative); the diagnosis is hereditary spherocytosis. This is a form of hereditary intravascular haemolysis where there is a defect in red cell membrane spectrin so that all are spherical in shape. The spleen recognises them as abnormal, and causes their destruction. Clinical sequelae include anaemia, splenomegaly, leg ulcers and pigment gallstones. Biochemical tests show a raised serum unconjugated bilirubin. The osmotic fragility test is most useful as osmotic fragility depends upon the volume to surface area ratio of the cells and reflects their ability to take up water without lysis. In normal red cells, the biconcave shape allows the cells to increase their volume by around 70% before lysis. In the spherocytic cell, the volume to surface area is increased, which limits the amount of water that can be taken up before lysis.

8 **Answer E:** This patient has von Willebrand disease, which is an abnormality of factor VIII, von Willebrand factor, and is usually inherited in an autosomal dominant manner. The disease is characterised by an increased bleeding time and reduced levels of factor VIII coagulant activity. Here there is no circulating antibody to factor VIII because there is a reduction of the APTT on mixing the plasma with normal plasma, the underlying cause being the reduction or structural abnormality of von Willebrand factor, which is needed to stabilise coagulation factor VIII and promote normal platelet function. He has a normal factor IX level, thereby excluding haemophilia B. There is no parent history here but the condition is autosomal dominant, and is one of the most common bleeding conditions. Most patients with mild disease respond to desmopressin (DDAVP), but clotting factor concentrates are needed for a minority.

9 **Answer B:** The clinical picture is of disseminated intravascular coagulation. When bleeding is the major problem, the aim is to maintain the prothrombin and active thromboplastin time at a ratio of 1.5 times the control, and the fibrinogen level above 1 g/L. Platelet transfusion is recommended if the count is less than $50 \times 10^9$/L. Anaemia is not very severe, so in this case fibrinogen replacement would be the appropriate choice.

10 **Answer E:** The classifications of sideroblastic anaemias are hereditary (congenital X-linked, AD, AR, mitochondrial cytopathy), acquired, as in myelodysplasia, drugs (such as ethanol, INH, chloramphenicol) and toxins (such as lead and zinc), and nutritional (including pyridoxine and copper deficiency).

**11 Answer D:** The diagnosis is heparin-induced thrombocytopaenia (HIT), and the new low platelet count is probably responsible for the purpuric rash. All anticoagulation should not be stopped, because of the risk of thrombotic complication. To commence warfarin is potentially hazardous, as warfarin inhibits protein C, and in the context of HIT, can precipitate venous limb gangrene or skin necrosis. The next management step is to commence hirudin, which is an inhibitor of thrombin.

**12 Answer A:** Tumour lysis syndrome from chemotherapy or massive cell lysis is the explanation of the electrolyte abnormalities.

**13 Answer D:** The cause of the patient's renal failure is hyperuricaemic nephropathy. The syndrome has previously been avoided by prophylactic allopurinol before and during chemotherapy, but the recombinant urate oxidase rasburicase may be better and is now licensed in haematological malignancies for the prophylaxis and treatment of hyperuricaemia.

**14 Answer E:** The side effects described are those of vincristine. Constipation and abdominal pain are common gastrointestinal side effects. Ataxia, loss of deep-tendon reflexes, foot drop and ataxia have been reported with continued administration. Other chemotherapy agents that cause neuropathy include platinum agents (cisplatin, oxaliplatin), taxanes (including paclitaxel and docetaxel) and other vinca alkaloids (vinblastine, vinorelbine).

**15 Answer A:** The best answer here is marrow suppression for chlorambucil therapy. Marrow infiltration by lymphoma is also possible. Widespread marrow infiltration in someone with low grade lymphoma is usually an end-stage feature. In this case, the blood film may demonstrate normoblasts and immature white cells. Hypersplenism may produce a pancytopaenia and can complicate any condition in which the spleen is enlarged. Anaemia of chronic disease or haemolysis may complicate lymphoma. However, this would not explain the low numbers of white cells and platelet count. In a patient with marrow suppression, the reticulocyte count alone is not a good guide to haemolysis.

**16 Answer A:** The patient presents with symptoms and signs of superior vena caval obstruction (SVCO). This is due to the anterior mediastinal mass and the single most useful diagnostic investigation is histological confirmation of the lesion from a biopsy. This can usually be done by a percutaneous CT guided biopsy. The most common cause of SVCO is primary lung cancer. Other causes include lymphoma. Treatment is of the underlying condition although in some cases of non-small cell lung cancer stenting of the SVCO may be required for relief of symptoms prior to chemotherapy/palliative radiotherapy. SVCO does not often need urgent treatment and the most important step is to obtain a histological diagnosis and then proceed with chemotherapy or radiotherapy. Steroids are often given; while there is no good evidence for their efficacy, they are helpful if there is stridor or if the diagnosis turns out to be lymphoma.

**17 Answer D:** This lady has hypercalcaemia, which is probably related to bony metastases secondary to breast carcinoma. The calcium is still elevated, despite adequate hydration with saline. The most appropriate next step is to give pamidronate, a bisphosphonate, to inhibit bone resorption and formation, thus reducing bone turnover. Many people are increasingly using the newer bisphosphonate zolendronic acid, which is considered better than pamidronate.

**18 Answer A:** The official answer is supposed to be option (A), but one has to acknowledge that pure choriocarcinoma is very rare, and usually in this rare disorder the HCG is much higher. The least unlikely differential diagnosis according to senior oncologists is MTU/MTT or non-seminomatous germ cell tumours (NSGCTs). (*See* **Learning point.**)

**19 Answer C:** Pathological fractures and bone pain are extremely common symptoms in patients with multiple myeloma. It is estimated that 70% of patients have bone pain at the time of presentation. Bisphosphonates reduce bony disease in myeloma, lowering the frequency of pathological fractures. There is also evidence that bisphosphonates modulate the disease and have some antitumour activity. As a result, bisphosphonates should be given routinely to patients with myeloma, even in the absence of hypercalcaemia.

**20 Answer E:** This elderly lady has metastatic gastric carcinoma and is dying. Her cancer is incurable, and she therefore needs to be kept pain-free. Treatment of the pneumonia is not appropriate, but she should be kept free from respiratory distress.

**21 Answer B:** The condition described is classical hereditary angioedema. This is typified by recurrent oedema, usually subcutaneous (non-itchy), laryngeal (stridor/airway obstruction), or intestinal (abdominal pain/vomiting). The onset is usually 1–2 hours, and resolution is usually within 24–48 hours. First attacks are usually in childhood, and precipitating factors include intercurrent infection, trauma, menstruation, and autoimmune disease (e.g. SLE). The most common finding is complement deficiency, with decreased inhibitor of activated C1, and there are two forms of the disease – decreased levels of C1 inhibitor (85%), and normal levels of C1 inhibitor but not functionally defective (15%). During an attack, C3 is normal and C2 and C4 are decreased. The rest of the options (apart from B) are true. Danazol or testosterone are used to prevent attacks, and treatment is with i.v. C1 inhibitor/FFP if unavailable, and aminocaproic acid.

22 **Answer B:** The history is strongly suggestive of systemic vasculitis, with mononeuritis multiplex, purpuric rash and haematuria. It is important to exclude conditions which can mimic vasculitis, such as infective endocarditis. The normal echocardiogram and negative blood cultures make this unlikely. Whilst polyarteritis nodosa can present with exactly this clinical picture, the marked consumption of C4, together with a strongly positive rheumatoid factor strongly suggests cryoglobulinaemia as the underlying cause. Cryoglobulins are immunoglobulins which precipitate in the cold. They can be type I (monoclonal; associated with lymphoproliferative disease), type II (mixed monoclonal and polyclonal), or type III (IgG polyclonal associated with immune complexes). Type I cryoglobulinaemia can be associated with many connective tissue disorders, chronic infections and most importantly chronic hepatitis C infection, which should always be excluded. Treatment of cryoglobulinaemia would include plasmapharesis, high dose steroids and cyclophosphamide.

23 **Answer B:** All the immunoglobulins are normal, apart from IgA, and the description fits. There is an association of this rare condition (1:500–700 incidence) with autoimmune syndromes such as rheumatoid arthritis, SLE, thyroiditis, pernicious anaemia, coeliac disease, and, associated with HLA B8, DR3. Treatment is with antibiotics.

24 **Answer B:** Angiotensin-converting enzyme inhibitors affect the metabolism of eicosanoids and polypeptides, including endogenous bradykinin. Patients receiving ACE inhibitors (including captopril) may be subject to a variety of adverse reactions, some of them serious. Angioedema involving the extremities, face, lips, mucous membranes, tongue, glottis or larynx has been seen in patients treated with ACE inhibitors, including captopril. Most cases occur within one week of starting therapy. If angioedema involves the tongue, glottis or larynx, airway obstruction may occur and be fatal. Emergency therapy, including but not necessarily limited to, subcutaneous administration of a 1:1000 solution of adrenaline should be promptly instituted.

# Learning Points

## *Question 1*

### Learning point

**Features of a sickle cell crisis**

Pain

Sickle cell anaemia (Hb SS) sometimes causes attacks of pain to the chest, abdomen, back, jaw, legs and arms. They occur because the 'sickling' of the red blood cells causes them to block up small blood vessels and stop the flow of blood. The sickling of red blood cells, which can cause a crisis, is more likely to take place under certain conditions. These include a reduction of the level of oxygen in the blood (after exertion, during anaesthetics or at very high altitudes), dehydration, and during pregnancy. Painful crises may also occur in association with febrile childhood or adult illnesses. If pain is very severe, admission to hospital may be necessary.

Anaemia

People with sickle cell disease are not always anaemic. In those with sickle cell anaemia, however, the haemoglobin is between 7 and 10 g/dL and the blood picture shows anisocytosis, sickle cells and a raised reticulocyte count due to haemolysis. The anaemia may become worse as a result of acute splenic sequestration or an aplastic crisis. If so, emergency treatment with blood transfusions may be necessary.

Infections

People with a sickle cell disorder are particularly prone to minor infections and also to serious and life-threatening infections like septicaemia, pneumococcal meningitis and osteomyelitis.

Other problems

Sickle cell disorders involve multiple systems. Children may get painful swelling of the hands and feet (called the hand-foot syndrome). They are also prone to enuresis and delayed puberty.

Adults (and sometimes children) can develop stiff and painful joints or ulcers on the lower legs. In general, people with sickle cell disease have an increased incidence of gallstones, jaundice, haematuria, strokes, priapism and difficulties during pregnancy and childbirth.

## *Question 3*

### Learning point

**Causes of a microangiopathic haemolytic anaemia (TTP or HUS)**

1 Infection (e.g. verocytotoxin-producing strains of *E. coli*, shigella, HIV)
2 Connective tissue disorders (SLE, scleroderma)
3 Malignant hypertension
4 Pregnancy
5 Malignancy (mainly adenocarcinoma)
6 Drugs (e.g. ticlodipine, oral contraceptive pill, ciclosporin)
7 Post-transplantation

HUS is characterised by microangiopathic haemolysis, thrombocytopaenia and acute renal failure. Clinically it is similar to TTP but neurological symptoms/signs are not a feature.

## *Question 18*

### Learning point

**Testicular tumours**

The classical presentation for testicular tumours is that of a healthy male in the third or fourth decade of life with a painless, swollen, hard testis. Testicular cancer can be divided into germ cell and non-germ cell tumours. Germ cell tumours are classified as either pure seminomas or mixed non-seminomatous germ cell tumours (NSGCTs): these two groups comprise more than 90% of all tumours. Non-germ cell malignancies (Leydig and Sertoli cell tumors, gonadoblastomas) make up less than 10% of all testicular tumors. Patients with history of cryptorchidism have a 10- to 40-times increased risk of testicular cancer and this risk is greater for the abdominal, versus inguinal, location of undescended testis. Orchidopexy does not reduce the risk of subsequently developing a malignancy. An abdominal testis is more likely to be seminoma, while a testis surgically brought to the scrotum by orchiopexy is more likely to be NSGCT. Choriocarcinoma is the most aggressive of the NSGCTs.

It disseminates hematogenously to lungs, liver, brain, bone, and other viscera very early in the disease process. Unlike classic seminoma or mixed GCTs, pure choriocarcinoma is more likely to present with symptoms from metastatic disease. Most testicular GCTs cause scrotal swelling, with a palpable mass. Choriocarcinoma is different, in that the local tumour may be small or nonpalpable. Pure seminomas do not cause a rise in AFP level (AFP is only produced by tumours containing embryonal and yolk sac elements). Elevated AFP levels are most consistent with NSGCT, though AFP is often within the reference range in pure choriocarcinoma.

HCG is usually markedly elevated in pure choriocarcinoma, but is only elevated in 10–15% of seminomas. Gynaecomastia occurs due to elevation of ßHCG levels and is therefore common in choriocarcinoma, but only rarely seen in patients with a seminoma. In ultrasound scanning, choriocarcinoma is associated with haemorrhage and necrosis and may appear more cystic, inhomogeneous, and calcified than a seminoma. Calcifications and cystic areas are less common in seminomas than in nonseminomatous tumours.

Urinary HCG, i.e. the pregnancy test, is an instant way to diagnose germ cell tumours in Casualty. In cases of metastatic disease, one should refer to an oncologist for consideration of emergency chemotherapy; since choriocarcinomas can have a doubling time of a few days, there is little point in asking the surgeons to perform an orchidectomy, which can however be done after the chemotherapy. Overall he would have a > 90% chance of being cured.

## *Question 19*

### Learning point

**Causes of increased susceptibility to fractures**

- Osteoporosis
- Hyperparathyroidism
- Metastatic carcinoma (especially breast, bronchus, prostate, kidney and thyroid)
- Leukaemia

## CHAPTER 3

# Dermatology

Dermatology is a broad topic, but generally pruritus, hyperpigmentation, erythema, loss of hair, trichosis, nail disorders, erythema nodosum and multiforme, purpura, vasculitis, psoriasis, urticaria, eczema, vitiligo, pemphigus and pemphigoid tend to be favourite topics.

# Questions

## Question 1

A 25-year-old man presents with a skin eruption affecting his face, scalp and chest. It has been deteriorating over the past few months. He is HIV-positive and is currently on zidovudine. On examination, he has a red, scaly eruption on his scalp, ears, nasolabial folds, and eyebrows. There are also dry, scaly areas in the presternal and interscapular areas, with extensive follicular papules.What is the most likely diagnosis?

A atopic eczema

B Kaposi's sarcoma

C rosacea

D seborrhoeic eczema

E psoriasis

## Question 2

Which of the following is not associated with neurofibromatosis type I?

A eight café au lait spots

B one plexiform neurofibroma

C three Lisch nodules

D sphenoid dysplasia

E acoustic neuroma

## Question 3

A 25-year-old man presents with non-pruritic white spots on his trunk. On examination, there are multiple sharply demarcated round hypopigmented macules of up to 2 cm in size, some of which appear to have coalesced. On gentle scratching, a delicate scaling is noted. There is no associated lymphadenopathy. There is no family history of depigmentation. Organisms are seen on direct microscopy, and under a Wood's lamp these lesions fluoresce with a pale greenish colour. The most likely diagnosis is:

A psoriasis

B pinta

C leprosy

D vitiligo

E pityriasis versicolor

## Question 4

A 36-year-old man presented with a three-week history of a rash on his abdomen and trunk. He first noticed a red, slightly pruritic lesion just to the left of his umbilicus several weeks ago. It was scaly and slightly raised. About seven days later, several similar but smaller lesions began to appear around the initial one. They continued to spread until they covered his entire abdomen and chest. On examination, there is a 3 cm × 1 cm oval lesion lateral to his umbilicus. The other lesions on his trunk appear the same except they are smaller. The most likely diagnosis is:

A tinea versicolor

B guttate psoriasis

C drug eruption

D pityriasis rosea

E secondary syphilis

## Question 5

A 45-year-old gardening enthusiast was referred to the Dermatology clinic with a well-circumscribed raised erythematous lesion on her finger. The lesion had enlarged steadily over the previous three weeks, was tender and bled easily when touched. The most likely diagnosis is:

A cutaneous anthrax

B keratoacanthoma

C malignant melanoma

D squamous cell carcinoma

E pyogenic granuloma

## Question 6

Which of the following is not commonly associated with drug-induced exacerbation of psoriasis?

A anti-malarial agents

B beta-blocking agents

C non-steroidal anti-inflammatory agents

D lithium

E thiazide diuretics

# Answers to Chapter 3: Dermatology

These solutions aim to provide the reason(s) for the right answer, and also the reason(s) for the wrong answers being excluded.

1 **Answer D:** Severe seborrhoeic eczema and seborrhoeic folliculitis are common in HIV infection, possibly due to an overgrowth of, or abnormal reactivity to *Malassezia* yeasts. The scalp, face, presternal area and interscapular regions typically are affected. HIV is also associated with Kaposi's sarcoma, which presents with red, brown or purplish macules, nodules or plaques and is associated with human herpes virus 8 infection. Herpes zoster typically presents with vesiculation.

2 **Answer E:** All of options A–D are associated with neurofibromatosis type I. D is an example of a distinctive osseous lesion; other examples include thinning of long bone cortex with or without pseudoarthroses. NF-1 is an autosomal dominant condition that shows complete penetrance and variable expression. It is caused by mutations in the NF1 gene in 17q11.2. Complications of this condition include learning difficulties, plexiform neurofibromas of the head and neck, scoliosis, hypertension, intracranial tumours and malignant change in cutaneous neurofibromas. Hypertension is seen in 5–6% of patients with NF-1, usually caused by renal artery stenosis or phaeochromocytoma, and the screening investigations in this patient should include 24-hour urinary VMA and catecholamine profile and plasma renin assay. Acoustic neuroma is associated with neurofibromatosis type 2, and may be confirmed by CT or MRI scan usually.

3 **Answer E:** The condition is pityriasis versicolor associated with the yeast *Malassezia*. The most appropriate antifungal treatment for pityriasis versicolor is to use a topical imidazole or terbinafine (Selsun). Alternative treatments include selenium sulphide lotion applied daily for 10–14 days.

4 **Answer D:** Pityriasis rosea is a self-limited, inflammatory dermatosis of unknown cause. It characteristically presents with oval, scaly, tannish-pink patches or plaques on the trunk, the generalised eruption being preceded by a single lesion ('herald' patch) by days to weeks. Typically, the lesions follow the skin cleavage lines. The lesions usually disappear within two months without any treatment.

5 **Answer E:** A pyogenic granuloma is a benign vascular lesion of the skin and mucosa, usually solitary in nature, often appearing as a glistening red papule or nodule that is prone to bleeding and ulceration. Lesions often grow rapidly over weeks, frequently at sites of trauma, and commonly involve the digits, arms, head and face. Keratoacanthoma is a rapidly growing nodular lesion with a central crater full of keratinous material. Clinically and pathologically

the lesions resemble squamous cell carcinoma. Cutaneous anthrax would not be expected on the basis of the history given. Anthrax lesions begin as reddened, indurated papules, later becoming necrotic with a characteristic black centre. Malignant melanomas may occur at any site, but most are pigmented. However, amelanotic melanoma is important in the differential diagnosis of pyogenic granuloma.

6 **Answer E:** The simple explanation is that all of the others can exacerbate existing psoriasis.

## CHAPTER 4

# Infectious diseases and tropical medicine

'Infectious diseases and tropical medicine' is another broad topic but relates to microbiology, treatment, and presentation of specific infections including:

- septicaemia
- meningitis/encephalitis
- endocarditis
- pneumonia
- tuberculosis
- PUO
- soft tissue infections
- intra-abdominal sepsis
- streptococcal infections
- gastrointestinal infections
- tropical infections including malaria, bilharzia, amoebiasis, filariasis, leishmaniasis, hookworm and viral haemorrhagic fevers
- viral hepatitis
- HIV/AIDS
- glandular fever syndrome and its differentiation from HIV seroconversion illness
- spirochaetosis–syphilis, borrelia (Lyme disease), and leptospirosis
- toxic shock syndrome and staphylococcal infections

# Questions

## Question 1

A 23-year-old woman, mother of three, developed anaphylaxis when she last received penicillin for orbital cellulitis. She re-appears to Casualty with a repeat episode of orbital cellulitis and cellulitis of her left shin.

The most appropriate antibiotic now is:

A cefuroxime

B gentamicin

C ciprofloxacin

D clindamycin

E meropenem

## Question 2

A 24-year-old student returns from a four month holiday trekking in Nepal. He had lost 12 kg in weight and had persistent watery and foul-smelling diarrhoea.

What organism is most likely to be the cause of his symptoms?

A *Cryptosporidium*

B *Entamoeba histolytica*

C *Giardia lamblia intestinalis*

D *Salmonella typhi*

E *Schistosoma mansoni*

## Question 3

A 27-year-old man presents with fever, urethritis and arthralgia. He has recently been on tour with his local football club, followed by a holiday to an island off Cyprus. He had enjoyed unprotected sexual intercourse whilst abroad, usually every morning. Shortly after his return to Heathrow Airport, he is found to have swollen knees bilaterally and left ankle, with a pustular rash on the dorsal aspect of his foot.

**Investigations revealed:**

**Blood tests:**

| | |
|---|---|
| haemoglobin | 15 g/L |
| white cell count | $16.2 \times 10^9$/L |
| neutrophils | $14.1 \times 10^9$/L |
| erythrocyte sedimentation rate | 65 mm/hr |
| rheumatoid factor | 10 iU/L |
| **Urinalysis:** | no cells, casts or bacteria seen. |

The most likely diagnosis is:

A gonococcal sepsis

B Lyme disease

C Reiter's syndrome

D staphylococcus arthritis

E tuberculous arthritis

## Question 4

A 31-year-old travel writer presented with pain in both ankles after a trip to Central America. He also complained of urinary frequency with suprapubic discomfort occurring two weeks previously while in Lima. He also had an acute fever, diarrhoea and abdominal pain. The stools did not contain blood or mucus and these symptoms settled in three days. He attributed it to some tribal food he ate but he denied consuming goat's milk. He also denied extramarital intercourse. Examination revealed an ill man with a temperature of 37.9°C, with mild bilateral conjunctivitis, a left-sided pleural rub and exquisitively tender ankle joints. There was also tenderness over the right iliac fossa but no palpable mass. Rectal examination was normal and sigmoidoscopy revealed some hyperaemia. Investigations revealed a normal blood film. Thick and thin films were performed three times to exclude malaria. The chest film was normal.

**Other investigations revealed:**

| | |
|---|---|
| haemoglobin | 12 g/L |
| erythocyte sedimentation rate | 80 mm/hr (Westergren) |
| white cell count | 14 × $10^9$/L (neutrophil leucocytosis picture) |
| serum sodium | 140 mmol/L |
| serum potassium | 3.4 mmol/L |
| serum bicarbonate | 30 mmol/L |
| serum creatinine | 100 µmol/L |

The most likely diagnosis is:

**A** gonococcal sepsis

**B** Lyme disease

**C** Reiter's syndrome

**D** staphylococcal arthritis

**E** tuberculous arthritis

## Question 5

An 80-year-old woman presents with confusion associated with a chest infection. She receives standard treatment, and four days later develops green, then bloody diarrhoea.

Which of the following organisms is likely to be responsible for her diarrhoea?

A *Campylobacter jejuni*

B *Clostridium difficile*

C *Escherichia coli* O157

D MRSA

E vancomycin-resistant *enterococcus*

## Question 6

Other than a mild sore throat in the preceding two days, a 19-year-old woman was completely well until some 12 hours prior to admission. She developed a severe headache with vomiting. On examination, she was febrile, pulse 38.1°C, BP 130/86. She had neck stiffness but Kernig's sign was negative. Her GCS was 15/15. There were no localising signs, and fundoscopy was normal. Careful examination of the skin revealed no rash, and the examination was also unremarkable. While waiting for her results, her GCS drops to 14/15 (E3, V5, M6).

The most appropriate therapy is:

A intravenous ceftriaxone

B intravenous ceftriaxone and dexamethasone

C intravenous ceftriaxone and aciclovir

D intravenous ceftriaxone, dexamethasone and aciclovir

E none of the above

## Questions 7 and 8

A 42-year-old woman is referred to the Outpatient clinic with a 7 year history of fatigue. She has also developed a rash over her lower legs. Ten years ago she underwent an abdominal hysterectomy which was complicated by post-operative haemorrhage. On examination, there is a palpable purpuric rash over both legs. Physical examination is otherwise normal.

**Investigations revealed:**

| | |
|---|---|
| haemoglobin | 13.1 g/L |
| white cell count | $9.0 \times 10^9$/L |
| platelet count | $212 \times 10^9$/L |
| serum sodium | 142 mmol/L |
| serum potassium | 4.2 mmol/L |
| serum urea | 8.5 mmol/L |
| serum creatinine | 81 µmol/L |
| serum total bilirubin | 6 µmol/L |
| serum alkaline phosphatase | 50 U/L |
| serum aspartate transaminase | 50 U/L |
| serum albumin | 42 g/L |
| rheumatoid factor | positive |
| complement C3 level | low |

Select the **two** most appropriate tests to secure the diagnosis:

A hepatitis C antibody

B HIV test

C cryoglobulins

D ANA

E anti-dsDNA antibody

F HLA typing

G radiolabelled white cell scan

H ultrasound of the abdomen

I laparoscopy

J erythrocyte sedimentation rate

## Question 9

A 45-year-old businessman presents with a six month history of weight loss, abdominal pain, and diarrhoea. His pain is intermittent, is associated with abdominal distension, and has been getting worse recently. He describes his stools as pale and difficult to flush away. He has lost 1 stone in weight despite eating reasonably well. He also has had recurrent fevers and sweats which can occur at any time. He travels frequently with his job and has recently returned from a two week trip to South Africa. His only other medical problem is transient migratory pains affecting his large joints, which he has had intermittently for the last five years and which do not seem to be getting any worse. He has been seen in the Rheumatology clinic but has recently been discharged without a diagnosis. He is found to be HLA B27 positive, and all his x-rays are reported as normal. His brother has a history of anterior uveitis. On examination, he appears anaemic and pigmented. He has signs of clubbing and enlarged cervical and axillary lymph nodes. His joints are normal. Other than a vague diffuse abdominal tenderness, examination of the abdomen is normal.

**Investigations revealed:**

**Blood tests:**

| | |
|---|---|
| haemoglobin | 10.4 g/L |
| MCV | 103 fL |
| white cell count | 8.4 × $10^9$/L |
| platelet count | 162 × $10^9$/L |
| erythrocyte sedimentation rate | 92 mm/hr |
| serum sodium | 137 mmol/L |
| serum potassium | 3.2 mmol/L |
| serum creatinine | 84 µmol/L |
| serum calcium (uncorrected) | 1.9 nmol/L |
| serum albumin | 24 g/L |

**Faeces:** negative for ova, cysts and parasites X 3

What is the treatment of choice?

A prednisolone and mesalazine

B cotrimoxazole and sulphamethoxazole

C gluten-free diet

D chloramphenicol

E prednisolone and nutritional supplementation

## Question 10

A 28-year-old woman was referred with jaundice, neck stiffness and headache. She also complained of red, gritty eyes. Her symptoms had started a week ago, as a 'flu-like illness', and had got progressively worse. She had just returned from a camping holiday in the USA in the Grand Canyon. There was no previous medical history and she was not on any medication apart from the oral contraceptive pill. She did not drink alcohol or smoke. She had, however, exactly three months previously been to a rather ethanolic leaving party for her best friend. On examination, she was jaundiced, and had bilateral suffuse conjunctivitis. Her temperature was 38.2°C, pulse 100 regular and blood pressure 120/90. Her JVP was not elevated, and her heart sounds and chest were clear to auscultation. There was some right upper quadrant tenderness, but no organomegaly. She was not encephalopathic. Kernig's sign was positive, but the rest of the neurological examination was entirely normal. There was no skin rash.

**Investigations revealed:**

**Blood tests:**

| | |
|---|---|
| haemoglobin | 11.7 g/L |
| white cell count | 12.3 × $10^9$/L (neutrophils 10.1, eosinophils 0.3, lymphocytes 1.9) |
| platelet count | 259 × $10^9$/L |
| serum sodium | 138 mmol/L |
| serum potassium | 4.9 mmol/L |
| serum urea | 5.8 mmol/L |
| serum creatinine | 70 µmol/L |
| serum albumin | 35 g/L |
| serum total bilirubin | 62 µmol/L |
| serum alanine aminotransferase | 148 U/L |
| serum alkaline phosphatase | 135 U/L |
| serum C-reactive protein | 200 g/L |

**Further tests:**

**Chest film (A-P):** lung fields normal; heart size normal.

The most likely diagnosis is:

A hepatitis A

B histoplasmosis

C leptospirosis

D Lyme disease

E Rocky Mountain spotted fever

## Question 11

A 28-year-old water-ski instructor was admitted as an emergency after collapsing at home. Other than a mild sore throat, he had been well until 12 hours prior to admission. He had an abrupt onset of feverishness, shivers, malaise, anorexia and vomiting, diarrhoea and increasing pain in his left thigh. On examination, he was flushed, unwell, and unable to stand. He had a temperature of 38.6°C, pulse 130 regular, JVP was not elevated, cardiac auscultation revealed an ejection systolic murmur at the left sternal edge. Chest was clear; respiratory rate was 24. The left thigh was exquisitely tender, but the overlying skin was normal other than a bruise following a minor injury at work. His hands and feet were warm, and peripheral pulses were present.

| **Blood tests:** | |
|---|---|
| haemoglobin | 15.4 g/L |
| white cell count | $18.5 \times 10^9$/L |
| platelet count | $91 \times 10^9$/L |
| serum sodium | 141 mmol/L |
| serum potassium | 3.9 mmol/L |
| serum urea | 9.5 mmol/L |
| serum creatinine | 138 µmol/L |
| serum total bilirubin | 20 µmol/L |
| serum alkaline phosphatase | 190 U/L |
| serum aspartate transaminase | 102 U/L |
| serum albumin | 32 g/L |
| **Chest film:** | clear |
| **Urinalysis:** | nil of note |

The most likely diagnosis is:

A necrotising fasciitis of the left thigh

B leptospirosis

C atypical pneumonia

D infective endocarditis

E infective enterocolitis

## Question 12

A 31-year-old Asian woman presented with a five-month history of lower abdominal pain, intermittent diarrhoea and weight loss of almost 8 kg. There was no blood in the stools. She was born in East Africa. Her parents migrated to England when she was aged 7. Since being in England, she had never been out of Europe. Both her grandfather and mother previously had tuberculosis. On examination, she was thin and pale. There was no clubbing. She had a temperature of 37.5°C. The abdomen was generally soft and tender. There was a palpable mass in the right iliac fossa. Rectal examination was normal. All other physical examination was normal.

**Investigations revealed:**

**Blood tests:**

| | |
|---|---|
| haemoglobin | 9.8 g/L |
| white cell count | $12.1 \times 10^9$/L |
| platelet count | $468 \times 10^9$/L |
| serum sodium | 139 mmol/L |
| serum potassium | 4.3 mmol/L |
| serum urea | 3.4 mmol/L |
| serum albumin | 33 g/L |
| erthyrocyte sedimentation rate | 66 mm/1st hr (Westergren) |
| serum C-reactive protein | 98 g/L |

**Further tests:**

| | |
|---|---|
| **Malarial (thick and thin films):** | negative |
| **Stool microscopy:** | no ova, cysts or parasites |
| **Chest x-ray:** | few calcified lymph nodes at the right hilum |

What is the most likely diagnosis?

- **A** Crohn's disease
- **B** ulcerative colitis
- **C** small bowel lymphoma
- **D** tuberculous ileitis
- **E** actinomycosis infection

## Question 13

A 23-year-old cocktail waitress was admitted as an emergency for pain over the right hypochrondium. The pain was worse on inspiration, Murphy's sign was negative and she began to vomit. Seven years ago, she had a casual sexual relationship and subsequently developed pustules all over the body, which cleared. Her male friend had a clear urethral discharge and arthritis of the right knee. On examination she was febrile at 37.6°C, breathless and tender over the right hypochrondium. A rub was audible over the liver, no organomegaly was detectable and she had a greyish white vaginal discharge. Her vital signs were normal and her symptoms subsided over the next few days while she was taking a course of antibiotics.

What is her most likely diagnosis?

A acute pancreatitis

B Fitz-Hugh-Curtis syndrome

C Crohn's disease

D tuberculous ileitis

E actinomycosis infection

## Question 14

A 17-year-old man, having just completed his GCSEs, is admitted with a 2 week history of fever, malaise, headache and night sweats. He has no cough, nor shortness of breath. He has some abdominal discomfort and back pain, but no bowel or urinary symptoms. His appetite is decreased, and he has just lost some weight. He has no other medical problems, and is on no other medication. Two months ago, he returned from Morocco, where he had stayed on his uncle's farm. On examination, he had cervical lymphadenopathy. His temperature was 37.8°C, pulse 99 (sinus rhythm), and blood pressure 90/65. Apart from hepatosplenomegaly (with no ascites), the rest of the clinical examination – including neurological examination – was entirely normal.

**Investigations revealed:**

**Blood tests:**

| | |
|---|---|
| haemoglobin | 11.7 g/L |
| white cell count | $3.0 \times 10^9$/L (neutrophils 1.6, eosinophils 0.2, lymphocytes 1.2) |
| platelet count | $150 \times 10^9$/L |
| serum sodium | 143 mmol/L |
| serum potassium | 4.3 mmol/L |
| serum urea | 3.5 mmol/L |
| serum creatinine | 65 μmol/L |
| serum albumin | 35 g/L |
| serum total bilirubin | 12 μmol/L |
| serum alanine aminotransferase | 37 iU/L |
| serum alkaline phosphatase | 120 U/L |
| erythrocyte sedimentation rate | 60 mm/hr (Westergren) |
| serum C-reactive protein | 48 g/L |

**Further tests:**

| | |
|---|---|
| **Malarial (thick and thin films):** | negative |
| **Chest x-ray:** | normal |

The most likely diagnosis is:

A brucellosis

B Hodgkin's lymphoma

C hydatid cyst

D schistosomiasis

E strongyloidiasis

## Question 15

The following syphilis serology results are from a 3-day-old baby and her 17-year-old mother. The baby has sticky eyes.

| | |
|---|---|
| Mother (from ante-natal clinic) | VDRL positive in 1:64<br>TPHA positive<br>FTA positive in 1:80 |
| Neonatal blood (taken on day 1) | VDRL positive in 1:32<br>TPHA positive<br>FTA positive (IgM positive at 1:40) |

What statement best fits with the syphilis serology above?

A baby has passive transfer of syphilitic antibodies from mother

B baby has active syphilis

C mother has had/still has syphilis

D both mother and baby are free from syphilis

E mother is immune from syphilis

## Question 16

As a medical registrar at a district hospital, you are called to see a 23-year-old Greek student who has just returned from a holiday in Thailand. He is markedly icteric, with diarrhoea.

**Investigations reveal:**

| | |
|---|---|
| haemoglobin | 9.7 g/L |
| white cell count | $5.6 \times 10^9$/L |
| platelet count | $87 \times 10^9$/L |
| serum C-reactive protein | 130 g/L |
| serum creatinine | 244 µmol/L |
| serum fibrinogen | 1.4 g/L |

Initial empirical therapy consists of intravenous ciprofloxacin, erythromycin and quinine. When you review the patient, he is markedly drowsy and hypotensive, with a widespread macular rash. What is the next best management step?

A give ceftriazone

B give intravenous saline

C perform a lumbar puncture

D check a BM

E refer immediately to a tertiary referral centre

## Question 17

A 45-year-old man appeared pale on returning from Asia after a stay of five years. During his stay, he had taken regular malaria prophylaxis. Three months after his return, he started to complain of weight loss, malaise and night sweats. On examination, his temperature was 38°C, pulse 90, BP 120/80. Small cervical lymph nodes and hepatosplenomegaly were noted (liver 5 cm below the costal margin, and spleen 10 cm below the costal margin). Investigations showed: serum haemoglobin 10 g/L, MCV 80 fL, white cell count $3 \times 10^9$/L (lymphocytes 70%, eosinophils 4%), platelet count $233 \times 10^9$/L, thick and thin films for malaria repeatedly negative. Serum urea 4 mmol/L, serum creatinine 110 µmol/L, serum albumin 30 g/L, and total protein 85 g/L. An HIV test was negative, Heaf test was grade II, and a plain chest x-ray was normal.

The most likely diagnosis is:

A Hodgkin's disease

B malaria

C tuberculosis

D visceral leishmaniasis

E brucellosis

## Question 18

A 52-year-old woman was admitted with malaise and leg weakness. Her illness started with a sore throat while travelling in Eastern Europe. On examination, she was febrile (39.1°C), with several areas of exudates on her pharynx and extensive cervical lymphadenopathy. There was weakness of the legs bilaterally with absent tendon reflexes.

What is the most likely diagnosis?

A acute myeloid leukaemia

B cytomegalovirus infection

C diphtheria

D glandular fever

E streptococcal tonsillitis

## Question 19

A 19-year-old woman presented with a 5 day history of fever, lethargy and cough followed by abdominal pain and frank haematuria. She had returned from Malawi a week ago, where she had been on safari. She had no other medical problems and had taken mefloquine malaria prophylaxis. She had one regular sexual partner and did not drink alcohol or smoke. Her temperature was 38°C, pulse 100 regular, and blood pressure 130/80. Physical examination was normal apart from cervical lymphadenopathy.

**Investigations revealed:**

| **Blood tests:** | |
|---|---|
| haemoglobin | 12.7 g/L |
| white cell count | $10.8 \times 10^9$/L (differential: neutrophils 8.3, eosinophils 1.1, lymphocytes 1.4) |
| platelet count | $219 \times 10^9$/L |
| serum sodium | 133 mmol/L |
| serum potassium | 5.2 mmol/L |
| serum urea | 12.8 mmol/L |
| serum creatinine | 200 µmol/L |
| serum total protein | 65 g/L |
| serum albumin | 35 g/L |
| serum total bilirubin | 12 µmol/L |
| serum alanine aminotransferase | 27 U/L |
| serum alkaline phosphatase | 120 U/L |

| **Further tests:** | |
|---|---|
| **Malarial (thick and thin films):** | negative |
| **Urinalysis:** | protein (+), blood (+++) |
| **Chest x-ray:** | patchy consolidation |

The most likely diagnosis is:

A blackwater fever

B brucellosis

C dengue haemorrhagic fever

D schistosomiasis

E typhoid

## Question 20

A 28-year-old man presented with a 1½ week history of fever, watery diarrhoea and abdominal pain, and now has developed a dry cough. He had returned from South Africa five days previously with his girlfriend, where he had been on safari. He had no previous medical problems, was on no medication, and did not take any form of malaria prophylaxis. On examination, he had a few cervical lymph nodes. His temperature was 39.0°C, pulse 64 regular, and blood pressure 118/76. JVP was + 2 cm, and heart sounds and chest were normal to auscultation. His abdomen was soft and he had 3 cm non-tender hepatomegaly.

**Investigations revealed:**

**Blood tests:**

| | |
|---|---|
| haemoglobin | 12.9 g/L |
| white cell count | $2.4 \times 10^9$/L (neutrophils 1.3, eosinophils 0.1, lymphocytes 1.0) |
| platelet count | $219 \times 10^9$/L |
| serum sodium | 139 mmol/L |
| serum potassium | 4.2 mmol/L |
| serum urea | 3.8 mmol/L |
| serum creatinine | 78 µmol/L |
| serum total protein | 65 g/L |
| serum albumin | 32 g/L |
| serum total bilirubin | 13 µmol/L |
| serum alanine aminotransferase | 25 U/L |
| serum alkaline phosphatase | 100 U/L |
| erythrocyte sedimentation rate | 36 mm/hr (Westergren) |
| serum C-reactive protein | 43 g/L |

**Further tests:**

| | |
|---|---|
| **Malarial (thick and thin) films:** | negative |
| **Urinalysis:** | negative |
| **Chest x-ray:** | normal |

The most likely diagnosis is:

A amoebic dysentery

B blackwater fever

C dengue haemorrhagic fever

D typhoid

E yellow fever

## Question 21

A 17-year-old Asian woman was admitted after collapsing at home. Although her family frequently travelled to India, she had not been abroad for two years. She had no significant past medical history, and was apparently completely well three hours prior to admission. On examination, she was profoundly shocked with an unrecordable blood pressure, pulse 78 regular. Jugular venous pressure was not elevated and heart sounds were normal. She was apyrexial, and the rest of the clinical examination was unremarkable.

**Investigations revealed:**

**Blood tests:**

| | |
|---|---|
| haemoglobin | 14.2 g/L |
| white cell count | $5.0 \times 10^9$/L |
| platelet count | $255 \times 10^9$/L |
| serum sodium | 137 mmol/L |
| serum potassium | 3.8 mmol/L |
| serum urea | 4.1 mmol/L |
| serum creatinine | 65 µmol/L |

**Further tests:**

| | |
|---|---|
| **Arterial gases, on air:** | pH 7.37, $pO_2$ 11.9, $pCO_2$ 5.1, oxygen saturations 96%. |
| **Chest film:** | normal |
| **ECG:** | QRS duration 0.16 s, PR interval 0.12 s. |

What is the most likely diagnosis?

A meningococcal septicaemia

B ruptured ectopic pregnancy

C chloroquine overdose

D anaphylaxis

E typhoid

## Question 22

A 24-year-old man presented with epistaxis, haematemesis and melaena for one day. Since arriving back in the UK from Burma five days ago, he had been having a flu-like illness associated with abdominal pain. He had taken malaria prophylaxis before he went. He had no significant previous medical history and was not on any medication except mefloquine. On examination, he looked unwell and jaundiced. There were non-blanching erythematous bruises on his skin. His temperature was 39°C, pulse 110 regular and blood pressure 96/64. Respiratory examination was normal. He had diffuse abdominal tenderness but no organomegaly or lymphadenopathy. Rectal examination revealed melaena.

**Investigations revealed:**

| **Blood tests:** | |
|---|---|
| haemoglobin | 11.1 g/L |
| white cell count | $2.8 \times 10^9$/L (nϕ1.4, eϕ 0.1, lc 1.1, mc 0.2) |
| platelet count | $99 \times 10^9$/L |
| serum sodium | 130 mmol/L |
| serum potassium | 5.2 mmol/L |
| serum urea | 12.8 mmol/L |
| serum creatinine | 228 μmol/L |
| serum albumin | 29 g/L |
| serum total bilirubin | 76 μmol/L |
| serum alkaline transferase | 85 U/L |
| serum alkaline phosphatase | 130 U/L |

| **Further tests:** | |
|---|---|
| **Malarial (thick and thin films):** | negative |
| **Urinalysis:** | protein (+++), blood (+++) |
| **Chest x-ray:** | normal |

The most likely diagnosis is:

A blackwater fever

B dengue haemorrhagic fever

C hepatitis A

D typhoid fever

E yellow fever

## Question 23

A 60-year-old farmer presents with a six-month history of recurrent night sweats and fever. He has lost approximately 5 kg in weight, and complains of fatigue. On examination, he is afebrile. Heart sounds are normal apart from a harsh ejection systolic murmur, a slightly displaced apex beat laterally, and his chest is clear. A spleen tip is palpable 4 cm below the left costal margin. The remainder of the examination is unremarkable, apart from a faint palpable purpuric rash around both ankles.

**Investigations reveal:**

| **Blood tests:** | |
|---|---|
| haemoglobin | 12.1 g/L |
| white cell count | $7.5 \times 10^9$/L |
| neutrophils | $5.5 \times 10^9$/L |
| lymphocytes | $2.0 \times 10^9$/L |
| monocytes | $0.05 \times 10^9$/L |
| eosinophils | $0.01 \times 10^9$/L |
| basophils | $0.01 \times 10^9$/L |
| platelet count | $114 \times 10^9$/L |
| serum aspartate transaminase | 98 U/L |
| serum alkaline phosphatase | 101 U/L |
| serum albumin | 39 g/L |
| serum sodium | 137 mmol/L |
| serum potassium | 4.2 mmol/L |
| serum urea | 9.3 mmol/L |
| serum creatinine | 170 µmol/L |
| serum total bilirubin | 12 µmol/L |

| **Further tests:** | |
|---|---|
| **Urinalysis:** | protein (+) |
| | microscopy: red cells, no bacteria |
| **Urine microscopy and culture:** | negative |

The most likely diagnosis is:

A brucellosis

B non-Hodgkin's lymphoma

C Q fever endocarditis

D renal cell carcinoma

E tuberculosis

## Question 24

Three months after a successful renal transplant, a patient presents with diarrhoea, arthralgia and fever. Serum creatinine is found to be 157 µmol/L, serum alanine aminotransferase 112 IU/L, white cell count $3.2 \times 10^9$/L, monospot negative. You see the same patient the following year in clinic. He again feels feverish and complains of a headache. The graft functions well on the new OKT3 antibody and tacrolimus. A lumbar puncture reveals: CSF lymphocytes 74/mm$^3$, protein 0.73 g/L, glucose 2.1 mmol/L, cryptococal antigen negative.

The best empirical therapy for this patient is:

A amphotericin

B rifabutin, clarithromycin and ethambutol

C ceftriaxone and ampicillin

D ceftriazone

E ganciclovir

## Question 25

A 75-year-old retired sheep farmer from Mid Wales is found to have mildly deranged LFTs during a routine health check-up prior to arranging his mortgage for his move to Birmingham, to become a farming executive. He has an ultrasound scan which demonstrates multiple cystic lesions in the right lobe of the liver ranging in size from 1–8 cm in diameter. The larger cysts have a calcified appearance. He had a melanoma removed from his back 20 years ago and has had multiple basal carcinomas removed from his head, face, and arms in recent years.

What is the next investigation?

A CT scan

B ERCP

C hydatid serology

D laparoscopy

E ultrasound-guided aspiration

## Question 26

A 19-year-old student was admitted with headache, photophobia and malaise for one day. She had no previous medical history and was not on any medication. On examination, she was drowsy and had a temperature of 38.5°C, pulse 110 regular, and blood pressure 90/55. JVP was +1 cm, and there was no focal neurological deficit. There was a non-blanching rash on her legs.

The **least** appropriate step in her immediate management is:

A inform consultant in charge of communicable diseases for tracing of close contacts

B intravenous aciclovir

C intravenous cefotaxime

D lumbar puncture, if clotting and platelet counts are normal

E nasal and throat swabs for microbiological analysis

## Question 27

A 48-year-old ex-professional tennis player returns from a European tournament early as he started abroad with abdominal pain, high fever, rigors and sweating. He is given cefotaxime by a doctor without effect. He now returns home to complain of a severe headache and right subcostal pain. On examination, he is pyrexial (39.2°C) and has some photophobia, but no neck stiffness. He is confused and disorientated, thinking he is still in Florence. Some small lymph nodes are palpable in the neck. He is tender in the right upper quadrant and some basal crackles are heard on one side.

**Investigations reveal:**

**Blood tests:**

| | |
|---|---|
| serum sodium | 123 mmol/L |
| haemoglobin | 12.9 g/L |
| white cell count | 11.8 × $10^9$/L |
| serum urea | 12.5 mmol/L |
| serum creatinine | 85 µmol/L |
| erythrocyte sedimentation rate | 28 mm/hr (Westergren) |
| serum total bilirubin | 12 µmol/L |
| serum asparate transferase | 499 U/L |
| serum alkaline phosphatase | 574 U/L |
| **Urinalysis:** | glucose (+), ketones (+), protein (+), blood (++) |

The next best treatment is:

A piperacillin

B cotrimoxazole

C teicoplanin

D erythromycin

E aciclovir

## Question 28

A 45-year-old lady went to West Africa on holiday, and then sustained an injury involving her head and abdomen. An emergency splenectomy was performed. Vaccines to the pneumococcus and meningoccus were given two weeks post-surgery to allow an antibody response to evolve, but obviously there had been no time for this patient to have been given any vaccines pre-operatively; nonetheless, it was considered by the doctors at the time that the immune response was sufficient. Investigations at the time show:

| | |
|---|---|
| haemoglobin | 6.5 g/L |
| platelet count | 270 × $10^9$/L |
| white cell count | 13.2 × $10^9$/L |

Liver function tests demonstrate an acute hepatitis. She is given an emergency blood transfusion. She returns four months later, and her blood pressure is then found to be 100/70, and her pulse is 136. Her temperature is 37°C, and she sustains a tonic-clonic convulsion. She is given anticonvulsants and antibiotics including penicillin V, but she appears jaundiced and is found to have a tender liver. On examination, she has 7 cm hepatomegaly. She is found to have night sweats and is found to be jaundiced, and there is a healed splenectomy scar.

What is the most likely cause of her jaundice?

A falciparum malaria

B amoebic liver abscess

C subphrenic abscess

D pneumococcal septicaemia

E transfusion-related hepatitis

## Question 29

A 35-year-old farmer presented with a tender itchy lesion on his right index finger that developed five days after feeding lambs. He had no other symptoms.

The most likely diagnosis is:

A anthrax

B herpetic whitlow

C molluscum contagiosum

D orf

E tinea manum

## Question 30

A 36-year-old farmer, recently returning from Morocco to visit his family in West London, presents with a fever and black malignant pustule on his right index finger. On examination, lymphadenopathy is also found.

The most likely diagnosis is:

A anthrax

B herpetic whitlow

C molluscum contagiosum

D orf

E tinea manum

## Question 31

A 62-year-old man presents with a dull aching pain in his left loin, a pyrexia, and haematuria. He gives a history of weight loss in excess of 5 kg over two months, and has had intermittent fevers during this time. There is no history of dysuria. He is an ex-smoker, and drinks less than 10 units of alcohol per week. Findings on examination include a pyrexia of 38.5°C, blood pressure 180/110. A left varicocoele is noted. The rest of the clinical examination is normal.

**Investigations revealed:**

**Blood tests:**

| | |
|---|---|
| haemoglobin | $18.5 \times 10^9$/L |
| white cell count | $14.0 \times 10^9$/L |
| neutrophils | $9.5 \times 10^9$/L |
| lymphocytes | $2.5 \times 10^9$/L |
| eosinophils | $0.9 \times 10^9$/L |
| platelet count | $420 \times 10^9$/L |
| erythrocyte sedimentation rate | 60 mm/hr (Westergren) |
| serum sodium | 140 mmol/L |
| serum potassium | 4 mmol/L |
| serum urea | 7 mmol/L |
| serum creatinine | 70 µmol/L |
| plasma glucose | 5.1 mmol/L |
| serum corrected calcium | 3.2 mmol/L |

**Further tests:**

| | |
|---|---|
| **MSU:** | RBC > 100, white cell count 10, no cells or casts, culture negative |
| **Blood cultures:** | X 4 negative after 72 hours |
| **Abdominal x-ray:** | calcification noted in the area of the kidney |

The most likely diagnosis is:

A hypernephroma

B perinephric abscess

C renal tuberculosis

D staghorn calculus (due to *Proteus* infection)

E Wegener's granulomatosis

## Question 32

A 67-year-old lady was admitted with a productive cough and confusion 10 days after being in hospital with a stroke. On examination, her temperature was 39°C. She had a residual left sided weakness but no other neurological deficit. Her pulse was 110 beats per minute and blood pressure 110/60 mmHg. Her respiratory rate was 22 breaths per minute. There was dullness to percussion at the right base with coarse crackles and an area of bronchial breathing. A chest x-ray revealed shadowing in the right lower lobe and a diagnosis of pneumonia was made. What is the most likely causative organism?

A anaerobic bacteria

B fungi

C Gram-negative bacteria

D Gram-positive bacteria

E legionella

## Question 33

Regarding pneumonia caused by *Legionella pneumophilia*, which of the following statements is **true**?

A it is associated with hyponatraemia

B it is best treated with intravenous amoxicillin and clavulanic acid

C it is common in AIDS patients

D it is readily diagnosed by standard aerobic sputum culture

E it should be managed on the ward in a respiratory isolation cubicle

# Answers to Chapter 4: Infectious diseases and tropical medicine

These solutions aim to provide the reason(s) for the right answer, and also the reason(s) for the wrong answers being excluded.

1 **Answer D:** Clindamycin avoids cross-reactivity, and is appropriate for the organism most likely to cause this clinical picture, which includes streptococcal Lancefield group 'A'. Clindamycin has been unfortunately maligned due to its association with pseudomembranous colitis. Although it is a bacteriostatic antibiotic, it acts by switching off protein synthesis within bacteria; this in turn will lead to decreased exotoxin expression, thereby removing the mediators of disease. Cefuroxime and meropenem are both b-lactams which have appreciable cross reactivity in respect of severe allergic reactions and should therefore be avoided. Streptococci are intrinsically resistant to gentamicin and ciprofloxacin.

2 **Answer C:** A severe Giardia infection is normally self-limiting after 7–14 days. Characteristic stools are loose, foul-smelling and often fatty. Positive diagnosis requires identification of cysts or trophozoites in stool specimens. Infections can be treated with a number of medications (e.g. metronidazole, tinidazole), but none is completely successful. Severe disease may persist longer and is debilitating.

3 **Answer A:** The most likely cause for his acute presentation is gonococcal septicaemia – with a pustular rash on the dorsum of his foot, fever, urethritis and oligoarthritis. The clinical picture is said to be typically a hot joint on a background of a migratory polyarthropathy. Reiter's syndrome is associated with an acute infection – urethritis/diarrhoea, and later the development of an arthritis. Disseminated disease is most common in women – men usually seek medical advice when urethritis develops because of severe pain. Conjunctivitis is common in Reiter's syndrome.

4 **Answer C:** Reiter's syndrome (reactive arthritis following an episode of dysentery). In post-dysenteric arthritis, the arthritis ocurs approximately two weeks after the initial symptoms. Weight-bearing joints are particularly affected asymmetrically and may have effusions. One should rule out gonococcal arthritis and there should be a diagnostic aspiration. The urethritis in Reiter's syndrome is usually mild. Ocular and skin involvement with pustular psoriasis of the solas (keratoderma blenorrhagica), circinate balanitis and pleurisy are rarer manifestations of the syndrome. The organisms usually implicated are *Shigella flexneri*, *Salmonella typhimurium*, *Yersinia enterocolita* and *Campylobacter*. Staphylococcal arthritis is most common in a previously damaged joint but may be associated with acute osteomyelitis. Lyme disease

may have a preceding rash associated with a tick bite, but is usually more chronic, TB is an osteomyelitis and chronic with other evidence of risk or exposure.

**5** **Answer B:** This is typical of *Clostridium* infection with pseudomembranous colitis induced by prior treatment with broad spectrum antibiotics such as cefuroxime, augmentin and the macrolides. It is treated with metronidazole as the first line treatment, and vancomycin as the second line treatment.

**6** **Answer B:** The diagnosis is meningitis, and the most suitable therapy empirically here is B.

**7, 8** **Answers A, C:** Hepatitis C antibody immunoassay will be required in part to secure the diagnosis of essential mixed cryoglobulinaemia (IgG and IgM), typically presenting with a vasculitic skin rash, Raynaud's phenomenon and a peripheral neuropathy.

**9** **Answer B:** The diagnosis is Whipple's disease, a multi-system disorder that is more common in people who are HLA-B27 positive. It usually presents as a malabsorption syndrome, but can also cause lymphadenopathy, hyperpigmentation and an arthropathy. More rarely, it may affect the central nervous system, lungs, heart or kidneys. A duodenal/jejunal biopsy is the investigation of choice, and infiltration of the section with macrophages which stain strongly with Periodic Acid Schiff and which contain intracellular bacilli (*Trophoryma whipelli*) is characteristic.

**10** **Answer C:** This patient presents with symptoms of jaundice, conjunctivitis, anaemia and meningism following the onset of a flu-like illness after a camping trip. During that time, she may have come into contact with contaminated water and contracted leptospirosis. If allowed to progress, it may lead to hepatic failure, meningitis and renal failure. There may occasionally be a rash but this is non-specific. Rocky Mountain spotted fever and Lyme disease are both associated with a characteristic rash, but do not cause liver dysfunction. Histoplasmosis may mimic tuberculosis but she has no chest signs, and a clear chest film. Hepatitis A does not usually cause conjunctivitis or meningitis.

**11** **Answer A:** For option B to be correct, one would expect a peripheral blood neutrophilia, against a background typically including lymphocytic meningitis. The history is typical of A. Necrotising fasciitis is included in the MRCP examination, as it is considered an emergency, with a mortality ranging from 20 to 50%. The process can progress very quickly in diabetics. A CT scan may demonstrate fascial oedema and tissue gas, but this should not delay surgical debridement rapidly. Anaerobes, enterobacteriaceae and streptococci may be involved, and ampicillin/gentamicin/metronidazole are reasonable.

12 **Answer D:** The diagnosis is tuberculous ileitis. The differential diagnosis is between tuberculous ileitis and Crohn's disease. Given the Asian race, TB ileitis is the most likely diagnosis. Other differentials include small bowel lymphoma, *Yersinia* enterocolitis and actinomycoses.

13 **Answer B:** The history is classical of Fitz-Hugh-Curtis syndrome (which is gonococcal or chlamydial perihepatitis). Adnexal tenderness is present on pelvic examination. There may be pain over the right shoulder. Other associated complications are endocarditis and PUO. One should perform a cervical swab for microscopy and culture, and perform chlamydial serology and blood culture. Ideally, smears for molecular diagnosis should be performed. Urine culture and microscopy should also be performed. The male partner should also be tested and treated, as the pustules and arthritis are highly suggestive of gonorrhoea.

14 **Answer A:** The long history of a 'flu-like illness, night sweats, pyrexia, cervical lymphadenopathy, and hepatospenomegaly after visiting a Mediterranean country is suggestive of brucellosis. The patient may have handled cattle, or ingested unpasteurised dairy products. Lymphoma is a possibility, but Hodgkin's disease would be more likely if there was associated eosinophilia and pruritus in an older person. Leishmaniasis is part of the differential diagnosis. The lack of eosinophilia excludes schistosomiasis and stronglyoides infection.

15 **Answer B:** The baby has active syphilis infection. There is evidence of active syphilis in the neonate rather than passive transfer of antibodies from the mother, as IgM is not transferred across the placenta (while IgG is).

16 **Answer D:** The answer is D because the likely diagnosis is severe falciparum malaria. Hypoglycaemia is a feature of malaria, and is made worse by the hyperinsulinaemic effect of quinine.

17 **Answer D:** The measure (total protein–albumin) gives a large immunoglobulin level, lending to answer D, but the clinical history is typical of visceral leishmaniasis. The causative agent is usually *Leishmania donovani*. The incubation period is very variable, ranging from two weeks to several months. Fever, malaise, weakness and weight loss are common. Hepatosplenomegaly develops gradually, and may be massive. With time, the skin develops a grey colour, and gives rise to the Indian name of the disease – kala-azar – meaning black fever. Anaemia is a common finding, and may be severe. Treatment is usually with pentavalent antimonial compounds.

18 **Answer C:** The history is of severe exudative pharyngitis against the background of E. Europe – highly suggestive of diphtheria, caused by *Corynebacterium diptheriae*, causing a severe pharyngitis with extensive soft tissue swelling and lymphadenitis 'bull-neck' appearance. Exotoxins produced

by the organism may cause myocarditis or neurological deficits. Neurology includes motor peripheral neuropathy.

19 **Answer D:** A patient with fever, haematuria, dry cough and eosinophilia should suggest a worm infestation. None of the other options is associated with eosinophilia > 0.4. The most likely organism is *Schistosoma haematobium*, contracted while swimming. Patients may also complain of pruritus and urticaria, diarrhoea, and have patchy consolidation on chest x-ray. Diagnosis involves microscopy of terminal urine, and treatment is with mebendazole.

20 **Answer D:** This patient has a persistent pyrexia, cough, altered bowel habit and abdominal pain without jaundice, which are all characteristic of typhoid. Rose spots tend not to develop until the second week of the illness. Dengue and yellow fever are viral haemorrhagic fevers, so jaundice and evidence of bleeding would be expected. Malaria is associated with low/normal neutrophil counts, but to develop blackwater fever one would expect a low platelet count suggestive of haemolysis. Amoebic dysentery is usually associated with an increased neutrophil count.

21 **Answer C:** Chloroquine overdose is the only explanation of the above, of all of the options provided, and around thirty tablets are apparently sufficient to kill a person. The clue is profound shock without a tachycardia. Drug overdose is likely here – tricyclic depressants would produce a tachycardia, dilated pupils and dry mouth. Chloroquine is a profound negative inotrope and chronotrope, and overdosage is treated with intravenous adrenaline and high doses of diazepam with respiratory support.

22 **Answer B:** Dengue fever is caused by an arthropod-borne flavivirus. It begins with symptoms of an upper respiratory tract infection. To diagnose dengue haemorrhagic fever there needs to be a fever of recent onset; dengue haemorrhagic fever has haemorrhagic manifestations, in this case headache, retro-orbital pain, musculoskeletal pain (severe pain is a feature), generalised lymphadenopathy, maculopapular ash, epistaxis, microscopic haematuria, haematemesis and melaena; low platelet count; and evidence of leaky capillaries, in this case serum albumin of less than 30. There is no available vaccination, and treatment is symptomatic. Yellow fever is another haemorrhagic fever, and has similar clinical features but is only found in Africa and South America, and a vaccination is available. Hepatitis A is unlikely, as the incubation period is normally 1–2 weeks and would be associated with more deranged transaminases in a patient who is this unwell.

23 **Answer C:** Q fever is a rickettsial zoonotic disease caused by *Coxiella burnetii*. Q fever is usually a self-limited respiratory illness due to the inhalation of infected aerosols, especially from animal products. Chronic infection may become established and can manifest as hepatitis, osteomyelitis or

endocarditis. The aortic valve is involved in over 80% of cases. Laboratory tests often show a hepatitis, anaemia, elevated erythrocyte sedimentation rate, thrombocytopaenia and hypergammaglobulinaemia. Microscopic haematuria may be present. The disease may be complicated by immune-complex mediated glomerulonephritis and arterial emboli. The diagnosis is best made serologically and phase I antibody titre to *Coxiella burnetii* (IgA and/or IgG) greater than 1/200 is virtually diagnostic of Q fever endocarditis.

**24** **Answer C:** Listeria is relatively infrequent as a cause of meningitis, but is common after renal transplant, especially in those with high dose immunosuppression. *Listeria monocytogenes* is a Gram-positive bacillus which commonly affects patients at the extremes of age and the immunosuppressed. CSF findings typically show a pleocytosis with a lymphocyte predominance. High dose ampicillin and ceftrixaone, or ampicillin and/or gentamicin are the treatment of choice.

**25** **Answer C:** Asymptomatic, calcified lesions in the liver are typical of hydatid cysts. Hydatid infection was endemic in sheep farming regions such as Wales or New Zealand in the past, and sheep dogs were infected by eating infected offal. Humans contract hydatids via faecal/oral spread from dogs. The liver cysts are usually asymptomatic and calcification usually denotes a non-viable cyst. Hydatid serology has a sensitivity of 80–90%. If this serology were negative, imaging +/- aspiration may be required.

**26** **Answer B:** This patient has bacterial meningitis, until proven otherwise. The most likely organisms are *Neisseria meningitides* or *Streptococcus pneumoniae.* Diagnostic tests that need to be taken include blood cultures, nasal and throat swabs for *N. meningidites* carriage, and serology and CSF for Gram stain. High dose intravenous antibiotics should not be delayed. Contact tracing is essential to ensure that close contacts are given antibiotic prophylaxis. There is nothing to suggest that she has encephalitis.

**27** **Answer D:** Legionnaire's disease usually starts with a non-specific prodrome, including fever, myalgias, malaise and headache. A temperature of 40°C (or higher) should be alerting. Almost 1/3 have pleuritic chest pain. A depressed mental state is frequent on admission. Hyponatraemia is seen in almost 40% of cases, and hepatic dysfunction manifested by abnormal liver enzyme levels and moderate increases in serum aminotransferase and serum total bilirubin levels are seen. Haematuria also occurs, and glomerulonephritis and pulmonary-renal syndrome has been described in some.

**28** **Answer B:** This is a rather confusing question, but the answer is B. 95% of amoebic liver abscesses present within five months of travel, and post-traumatic splenectomy is considered to be a risk factor.

**29 Answer D:** Orf or ecthyma contagiosum is a viral infection which begins as an inflamed reddened papule that may enlarge to form a nodule that often resolves spontaneously. It is associated with contact with infected sheep, especially lambs. Anthrax is a bacterial infection discussed later in this chapter.

**30 Answer A:** Anthrax has an incubation period of 1–7 days. It is a Gram positive rod diagnosed in cultures from skin or nasal swabs or blood cultures. Three forms of disease include cutaneous (95%), pulmonary and ingestion. Cutaneous anthrax results in a black eschar (malignant pustule) 4–9 days after exposure. Oedema, fever and hepatosplenomegaly may also be present. Only those directly exposed to spores should be given 60 days of oral ciprofloxacin 500 mg bd. Chest x-ray findings with pulmonary anthrax include widened mediastinum, lymphadenopathy and haemorrhagic mediastinitis. These findings can also occur with tuberculosis. The prognosis is poor. Anthrax has two forms: cutaneous and respiratory. This is clearly a case of cutaneous anthrax.

**31 Answer A:** The question is to emphasize that a patient with a fever does not necessarily indicate that the question involves infectious diseases. Please be reminded that the questions are randomized in the actual examination, regarding the topic covered, and are ***not*** introduced with topic headings. Males > female = 2:1 ratio. Classically presents with the triad of haematuria, loin pain and swelling. Seldom presents with all three symptoms. Associated with hypertension and high-output cardiac failure. The tumour is associated with increased production of erythropoietin and possible occlusion of the renal vein causing a varicocoele. The majority of these tumours are now diagnosed on ultrasound. The metastases (cannonball to the lung and lytic to the bone) are also very vascular, and single chest metastases may be resected. Treatment is by surgical resection–renal artery embolisation pre-operatively. 5 year survival is 30–50%.

**32 Answer C:** With a pneumonia occurring so soon after discharge from hospital, this lady should be treated as having a (late) hospital-acquired pneumonia. Her age and recent CVA are risk factors. The most common organisms are Gram-negative bacteria although anaerobic bacteria are common, particularly if there is a history of aspiration.

**33 Answer A:** This is more of a Part 1 type question, but is included here as a learning point. *Legionella pneumophilia* is a Gram-negative bacillus that is ubiquitous in the environment. It is an example of an 'atypical' pneumonia. The prodrome normally consists of malaise, myalgia, and headache. A useful rapid confirmatory test is the urinary *Legionella* antigen, although sputum cultures may be of use. Erythromycin/clarithromycin are considered by some as the antibiotics of choice but the MRCP examination considers as acceptable a macrolide (erythromycin or clarithromycin), and rifampicin; alternatives include doxycycline, cotrimoxazole or ciprofloxacin. The chest x-ray appearance of legionnaire's disease can vary widely from a ground-glass appearance to a peripheral lobar consolidation. Deranged liver enzymes are common; it may be associated with outbreaks but sporadic cases are common. (*See* **Learning point**.)

# Learning Points

## *Question 33*

### Learning point

**Atypical pneumonias**

- Difficult to grow in culture
- Extrapulmonary features often
- Odd blood tests often
- Diffuse CXR changes

Human infection occurs when a sufficient inoculum of bacteria are aerosolised and inhaled. A variety of environmental sources have been identified as reservoirs of *Legionella* and have been responsible for infection in humans, including air conditioners, humidifiers, shower units and jacuzzis. *Legionellae* do not grow on standard culture media, but require specific supplemented media; they grow best at a low pH. *Legionella* pneumonia is more common in men than in women, by a ratio of about 3:1. Other factors that predispose to infection include smoking, alcoholism, old age, chronic illness and immunosuppressive therapy (although it is not more common in AIDS). Typically, the history is of recent foreign travel, cough, gastrointestinal symptoms, deranged liver function tests (usually a transaminitis), and a right upper lobe pneumonia; the patient often presents with confusion, which may represent a toxic encephalopathy.

# CHAPTER 5

# Rheumatology

Rheumatology is concerned with the science behind the presentation, investigations, and management of common conditions for the MRCP. Common conditions are reflected in the frequency of their questions, i.e. inflammatory arthritis, back pain, periarticular disorders, osteoarthritis, connective tissue diseases, and bone diseases. However, all candidates must be able to answer questions on the management of acute rheumatological emergencies, including septic arthritis, osteomyelitis, temporal arteritis and acute spinal cord compression.

## NORMAL VALUES (BLOOD)

| | | |
|---|---|---|
| complement component C3 | | 60–180 mg/L |
| complement component C4 | | 10–35 mg/L |
| immunoglobulins | IgG | 6–13 g/L |
| | IgA | 0.8–3.7 g/L |
| | IgM | 0.4–2.2 g/L |

# Questions

## Question 1

A 67-year-old man, on steroids, with a known diagnosis of rheumatoid arthritis, presents with a week's onset of an unilateral left-sided knee effusion. He has noticed some night sweats, and the loss of 2 kg of weight over a month. The knee is minimally painful. Investigations include a low grade neutrophilia, erythrocyte sedimentation rate of 40 mm/hr (Westergren). An aspirate of synovial fluid appears purulent. X-ray of the knee demonstrates subchondral cysts and severe loss of bone.

The next best investigation to confirm the diagnosis is:

A synovial fluid culture

B rheumatoid factor

C culture of synovial tissue biopsy

D microscopy of synovial fluid for acid-fast bacilli

E microscopy of synovial fluid for crystals

## Question 2

A 73-year-old male presented with an acute attack of gout in his left knee.

What is the most likely underlying metabolic cause?

A decreased renal excretion of uric acid

B overproduction of uric acid

C excessive dietary purine intake

D lactic acidosis

E starvation

## Questions 3 and 4

An otherwise fit 68-year-old, but rather obese, woman complained of pain at the base of her right thumb, as well as pain in both of her knees. The pain is worse on walking, and there is marked morning stiffness for about 10 minutes. She reported no difficulties in using her wrists in daily activities. Previous medical history was unremarkable, and her health, including her renal function, was entirely normal otherwise. Social history elicited that her diet was good, and she was still attending the gym to try the treadmill at her leisure. On clinical examination, there was tenderness and swelling of the right first carpometacarpal joint and of both knees bilaterally. Moderate crepitus was found.

## Question 3

The most likely diagnosis is:

A avascular necrosis of the scaphoid

B De Quervain's tenosynovitis

C osteoarthritis

D psoriatic arthritis

E rheumatoid arthritis

## Question 4

What is the best treatment?

A celecoxib

B naproxen

C dihydrocodeine

D paracetamol

E topical diclofenac

## Question 5

A 24-year-old Turkish woman has recently gained employment as a checkout assistant at her local supermarket, but is referred by her employer with tiredness. She reports to her general practitioner a history of intermittent blood diarrhoea, and a history of cerebral venous thrombosis. On examination, the sclera of the right eye is inflamed, and multiple mouth ulcers are noted. At colonoscopy, which confirmed colitis, two large vulval ulcers were noted.

Which of the following skin manifestations would be unlikely in this lady?

A erythema nodosum

B thrombophlebitis

C acneiform skin eruption

D pathergy

E livedo reticularis

## Question 6

A 24-year-old English man was referred because of a 5 month history of lower back pain, radiating to his buttocks, and back stiffness worse in the morning and after periods of inactivity, but which improves with exercise. Erythrocyte sedimentation rate is 38 mm/hour. X-rays of the sacroiliac joints are normal.

The most likely clinical sign is:

A restricted straight leg raising

B positive Trendelenburg test

C positive femoral stretch test

D exaggerated lumbar lordosis

E sacroiliac joint tenderness

## Question 7

A 32-year-old previously well female presents with a seven month history of pain and stiffness in her joints. Examination reveals synovitis of the distal interphalangeal joints of the left index finger, and the right ring finger, together with the left wrist and left ankle joints. The erythrocyte sedimentation rate is 35 mm in the first hour.

Which one of the following is the most likely diagnosis?

A osteoarthritis

B psoriatic arthritis

C rheumatoid arthritis

D systemic lupus erythematosus

E viral arthritis

## Question 8

A 51-year-old female is referred by her GP over concerns about osteoporosis. She had a hysterectomy and oophorectomy because of uterine fibroids one year ago, after which she developed hot flushes that persist. Her elderly mother recently fractured the neck of her femur and the patient is worried about the possibility that she too will fracture her hip later in life. She is otherwise well, is a non-smoker, drinks about five units of alcohol weekly and has a healthy diet. Examination reveals a fit thin female with a BMI of 18. Her blood pressure is 122/88 mmHg and breast examination is normal.

Which of the following would you recommend for her?

A bisphosphonates

B calcitonin

C combined oestrogen and progesterone therapy

D unopposed continuous oestrogen therapy

E vitamin D supplements

## Question 9

A 65-year-old woman presents with a one month history of malaise, weight loss and right sided pain around the eye. She has noticed headaches and intermittent diplopia. Five years previously, she had a mastectomy for carcinoma of the breast. On examination, her temperature was 37.5°C, there was scalp tenderness and tenderness of the right forehead and temple. There was some weakness of abduction of the right eye, and some subtle bilateral proximal myopathy was noticed.

**Investigations revealed:**

erythrocyte sedimentation rate (Westergren) 55 mm/hr
Nil else

The most likely diagnosis is:

A conversion disorder

B thyroid eye disease

C giant cell arteritis

D meningeal metastatic disease

E posterior communicating artery aneurysm

## Questions 10 and 11

A 35-year-old woman with newly diagnosed rheumatoid arthritis would like some information from you regarding her prognosis. Which two features from the list below are the best predictors of subsequent disability and joint damage in rheumatoid arthritis?

Select 2 of the following features:

A anti-cyclic citrullinated peptide antibody

B female sex

C rheumatoid factor positivity

D HLA DR3 genetic marker

E poor functional status at presentation

F high educational level

G presence of nodules

H negative ANA

I insidious onset of arthritis

J erythrocyte sedimentation rate of 33 mm/hr (Westergren)

## Question 12

A 35-year-old female complains of a five year history of widespread muscle and joint pain, fatigue and poor sleep. Examination is normal, except bilateral tender spots in the occipital region, trapezius muscles, rhomboid muscles, lateral epicondyles of the elbows, low back and gluteals are noted. All blood tests, including erythrocyte sedimentation rate, thyroid function tests, and creatinine phosphokinase, are normal.

The most likely diagnosis is:

A rheumatoid arthritis

B polymyositis

C fibromyalgia

D systemic lupus erythematosus

E reactive arthritis

## Question 13

A 22-year-old nursery school teacher is referred to clinic by her GP. She gives several weeks' history of swollen, tender finger joints. She has no previous medical or surgical history of note, and has been entirely well apart from feeling fatigued for a few days recently. The only sick contacts she could recall were several of the children in her class who had been recently off sick with a mild self-limiting illness, consisting of a fever, rhinorrhoea and a rash. On examination, the metacarpophalangeal joints and proximal interphalangeal joints of both hands are swollen and tender. Serology is unavailable, and complement levels C3 and C4 are quite low.

What do you think is the most likely diagnosis?

A adult Still's disease

B Lyme disease

C parvovirus B19 infection

D rheumatoid disease

E systemic lupus erythematosus

## Question 14

Which of the following clinical features is unusual in adult onset Still's disease?

A arthralgia

B lung fibrosis

C fever

D pericarditis

E splenomegaly

## Question 15

Which of the following features is most suggestive of serious pathology in a 67-year-old man presenting with low back pain?

A long history of back pain

B pain which wakes the patient at night

C pain on movement

D a history of minor trauma

E severity of pain

## Question 16

A patient of yours attends your general medical clinic, presenting her 9-year-old girl with arthralgia affecting the small joints of her hands and feet, and increasing difficulty in mobilising. The Gower's manoeuvre is abnormal. There is oedema around the eyelids and face, an ulcerated rash over the extensor surfaces of the fingers, elbows, knees and ankles, and periungual telangiectasia.

What is the most likely diagnosis?

A scleroderma

B Kawasaki disease

C juvenile dermatomyositis (JDMS)

D systemic lupus erythematosus

E psoriasis

## Question 17

An otherwise fit 69-year-old woman was admitted following attendance at Casualty, for recent onset of deafness. Systematic enquiry, aside from diffuse 'aches and pains', is entirely unremarkable. Investigations:

**Blood tests:**

| | |
|---|---|
| serum albumin | 38 g/L |
| serum total protein | 78 g/L |
| serum aspartate transaminase | 20 U/L |
| serum alanine aminotransferase | 39 U/L |
| serum lactate dehydrogenase | 220 U/L |
| serum alkaline phosphatase | 280 U/L |
| serum gamma glutamyl transferase | 28 U/L |
| serum total bilirubin | 14 μmol/L |

**Further neurological tests:**

| **Rinne's test** | **Left ear** | **Right ear** |
|---|---|---|
| air conduction | + | +++ |
| bone conduction | + | + |
| **Weber's test** | + | ++ |

+ represents intensity.

The most likely diagnosis is:

A earwax

B cerebellopontine lesion (such as acoustic neuroma)

C polymyalgia rheumatica

D Paget's disease

E metastases of a primary cancer, most likely breast

# Answers to Chapter 5: Rheumatology

These solutions aim to provide the reason(s) for the right answer, and also the reason(s) for the wrong answers being excluded.

1 **Answer C:** The patient is already known to have rheumatoid arthritis, and therefore the use of rheumatoid factor is of little use now. This is a difficult question, instead, about tuberculous arthritis, and this man is at risk because of his diagnosis of rheumatoid disease and the fact that he is on steroids. Other risk groups include the immigrant population, especially Asian, and the iatrogenically immunosuppressed, e.g. on cancer chemotherapy regimes. The Mantoux test is often negative, whilst the erythrocyte sedimentation rate is invariably elevated. Routine microscopy for acid-fast bacilli is often negative, as is culture. Synovial biopsy, or synovectomy, is diagnostically much more reliable, often revealing typical cavitating granulomas around which acid-fast bacilli may be identified. The most striking radiological feature of tuberculous arthritis is the involvement of juxta-articular bone. Subchondral cysts are common and loss of bone may be severe.

2 **Answer A:** The aetiology of gout can be broadly divided into cases where there is underexcretion of urate via the kidney (90%) or endogenous overproduction of uric acid (10%), although the distinction is rarely of therapeutic benefit, as allopurinol (which reduces the concentration of urate in blood and urine) is the mainstay of treatment. In a 73-year-old man, it is almost certainly reduced renal excretion due to deteriorating renal function and possibly thiazide diuretic use.

3 **Answer C:** Osteoarthritis of the 1st carpometacarpal joint is extremely common in a 68-year-old lady and is the most likely diagnosis. Swelling is usually bony hard and due to osteophyte formation, which can lead to the appearance of squaring of the hand. De Quervain's tenosynovitis is a common overuse condition indeed does present with pain or tenderness at the base of the thumb, and usually is associated with discomfort on using the wrist. As for the correct option, obesity is an obvious risk factor. Crepitus is a grinding noise made by irregular cartilage moving over a similar surface.

4 **Answer D:** The recommendations of the American College of Rheumatology, published in *Arthritis and Rheumatism* (2000), recommended acetaminophen (paracetamol) together with non-pharmacological interventions (exercise, diet) as first line therapy of mild/moderate OA of hips and knees. Naproxen is a NSAID, and, as such, a preventable cause of mortality and morbidity from upper GI bleeding; currently there is a considerable debate about the role of the COX-2 inhibitors such as celebrex in this condition.

5 **Answer E:** The description is classic of Behcet's syndrome, with oral and genital ulceration, colitis and scleritis. Behcet's syndrome is also typified by eye lesions, arthritis and skin lesions, including erythema nodosum, thrombophlebitis, acneiform skin eruptions, and pathergy (hyperirritability of the skin). This condition is more prevalent from the Eastern Meditteranean and Turkey to the Far East and there is an association with HLA-B5 and HLA B51. 25% of patients may develop arterial or venous thrombosis, which may lead to the formation of aneurysms. Up to 1/3 of these patients may have the factor V Leiden mutation. Livedo reticularis is classically associated with antiphospholipid syndrome. Positive test is > 2 mm erythema, 24–48 hours after a 25 gauge needle is pricked to a depth of 5 mm.

6 **Answer E:** This is a common presentation of ankylosing spondylitis. MRI of the sacroiliac joints as well as x-ray of the lumbo-sacral spine may be suitable investigations to establish this diagnosis. Early sacroiliitis has a 'rosary bead' appearance. One may see early changes such as Romanus lesions and squaring of the vertebral bodies. HLA B27 is present in over 90% of white AS patients, but the prevalence is 8% in healthy whites, and hence the test is not diagnostic.

7 **Answer B:** The lengthy history with an oligoarticular involvement, but affecting the distal interphalangeal joints, despite the lack of any previous history of psoriasis, is highly suggestive of psoriatic arthropathy. The synovitis would argue against a diagnosis of osteoarthritis, and the absence of any other supportive features (rash) makes SLE unlikely. One would expect a more symmetrical arthropathy, with rheumatoid arthritis, and it has progressed way beyond the acute period expected for viral arthritis.

8 **Answer D:** This patient has a risk for osteoporosis, being thin and recently having had an oophrectomy. Current guidelines recommend the use of oestrogen replacement as first-line therapy in such patients. Unopposed oestrogen therapy is most appropriate as the patient has had a hysterectomy and combined HRT is unnecessary. Tibolone, raloxifene and bisphosphonates are recommended as second line agents where HRT may be poorly tolerated or contraindicated. Although things are continuing to change, with regard to publications such as the *Women's Health Study* and the *Million Women Study*, the fact remains that in symptomatic patients, HRT offers the best therapeutic option and in the absence of any cardiovascular risk factors, is recommended. HRT remains the first-line therapy for treatment of peri-menopausal symptoms such as hot flushes and conveys some protective benefit for bones during the early postmenopause. This choice should be reconsidered after 3–5 years, when bone protection becomes the most pertinent issue and the risk of breast cancer is beginning to increase. At this point a DEXA scan should be performed and specific bone therapy considered.

9 **Answer C:** The description is classical for giant cell arteritis, and should be always considered in patients with headaches, ocular symptoms, systemic symptoms and a raised erythrocyte sedimentation rate. The erythrocyte sedimentation rate is almost always > 50 mm/hr at presentation, however may have returned to normal after five days of prednisolone therapy. The specificity of raised erythrocyte sedimentation rate is < 50%. Temporal artery biopsy remains the gold standard, and is positive up to 14 days after initiation of steroid therapy. One should try to get a biopsy as soon as possible, without delaying steroid treatment.

10/11 **Answers C, E:** Factors C and E are very important in this context, and best predictors of subsequent disability and joint damage. HLA DR4 incidentally is associated with worse prognosis. Extra-articular manifestations, including nodules and vasculitis, low educational level, 30% ANA positivity, acute onset, and persistently elevated erythrocyte sedimentation rate are associated with a poor outcome.

12 **Answer C:** The long history, with multiple tender joints in characteristic locations and normal investigations, confirms fibromyalgia. This is actually a diagnosis of exclusion.

13 **Answer C:** The most likely diagnosis is parvovirus infection. (*See* **Learning point**.)

14 **Answer B:** The order is (roughly) arthralgias (98–100%), fever (83–100%), myalgias (84–98%), sore throat (50–92%), rash (87–90%), lymphadenopathy (48–74%), splenomegaly (45–55%), hepatomegaly (29–44%), pericarditis (24–37%), and pneumonitis (9–31%). (*See* **Learning point**.)

15 **Answer B:** 95% of lower back pain is mechanical/degenerative in nature. Clinical red flags suggest more serious pathology, such as cancer or infection, and require further investigation. Age onset < 20, > 55, constant, progressive pain at night, thoracic pain, systemically unwell, weight loss, neurological signs, and raised erythrocyte sedimentation rate are all poor prognostic signs according to the Clinical Standards Advisory Group guidelines, 1984.

16 **Answer C:** JDMS is a myositis with a characteristic skin rash and vasculitis. The periorbital heliotrope rash can be associated with oedema and the Gottron's papules on the extensor surfaces may ulcerate. The myopathy is proximal and arthritis can occur in a third of cases. The muscle enzymes can be normal. There is no association with underlying malignancy. Ectopic calcification may be seen in the tissues.

17 **Answer D:** The aetiology of an isolated serum alkaline phosphatase, of bone origin, in a 68-year-old with recent onset sensorineural deafness suggests the diagnosis of Paget's disease. Secondary carcinoma, however, should be

excluded. Common complications of Paget's disease include high-output cardiac failure, osteosarcoma, bone pain, secondary osteoarthritis, pathological fracture.

# Learning Points

## *Question 13*

### Learning point

**Parvovirus (B19) infection**

Parvovirus B19 infection may also be associated with a symmetrical post-infectious arthritis, affecting the small joints of the hands, wrists, and feet. The knees or elbows are rarely involved. The arthritis is much more common in adults, particularly in women, and may persist for weeks to months (even years in a small number of patients). The arthritis may mimic rheumatoid arthritis, and, like rheumatoid arthritis, joints on both sides of the body are usually affected. Unlike rheumatoid arthritis, the postinfectious arthritis associated with parvovirus B19 does not cause permanent damage to bones or joints. Weakly positive serology is not unusual, and there may be hypocomplementaemia. If IgM antibody to parvovirus B19 is detected, the test result suggests that the person has had a recent infection.

## *Question 14*

### Learning point

**Diagnostic criteria for systemic juvenile chronic arthritis (the childhood form of adult onset Still's disease)**

1 Daily fever > 39°C
2 Arthralgia or arthritis
3 Absence of rheumatoid factor
4 Absence of ANA

Plus two of the following: a) leucocytosis > $15 \times 10^9$/L, b) maculopapular rash, c) serositis, d) hepatomegaly, e) splenomegaly, and f) generalised lymphadenopathy.

# CHAPTER 6

# Clinical pharmacology and toxicology

Broadly speaking, this section of the written paper examines the need for monitoring of routine drug therapy, important drug interactions, and therapeutics for specific patient groups such as the elderly, pregnancy, patients with renal disease, and patients with hepatic disease. Clinical toxicology is a major focus of the examination, and examples of question topics may include poisoning connected with: paracetamol, salicylate, tricyclic antidepressants, lithium, iron, digoxin, and drugs of abuse (DOA).

## THERAPEUTIC DRUG LEVELS

| | |
|---|---|
| plasma aminophylline | 10–20 μg/mL |
| plasma carbamazepine | 34–51 μmol/L |
| blood ciclosporin | 100–150 nmol/L |
| plasma digoxin (taken at least 6h post dose) | 1–2 nmol/L |
| plasma ethosuximide | 280–710 μmol/L |
| blood gentamicin (peak) | 5–7 μg/mL |
| serum lithium | 0.5–1.5 mmol/L |
| serum phenobarbital | 65–172 μmol/L |
| serum phenytoin | 40–80 μmol/L |
| serum primidone | 23–55 μmol/L |
| plasma theophylline | 55–110 μmol/L |

# Questions

## Question 1

A 74-year-old female presents as a first acute admission with confusion and diarrhoea. Little is known of her past medical history except that it is noted on the GP letter that she is receiving treatment for manic depression and hypothyroidism. Examination reveals that she has a Glasgow Coma Scale of 14 but is confused. She is thin, unkempt and dehydrated with a temperature of 37°C. She has a pulse of 82 beats per minute in a regular rhythm and a blood pressure of 112/72 mmHg. She is noted to have a coarse tremor and dysarthric speech.

Which of the following do you think is the most appropriate investigation to assist in her management?

A arterial blood gas analysis

B CT scan of the head

C serum lithium measurement

D serum electrolytes

E thyroid function test

## Question 2

A 46-year-old is admitted and found to have paracetamol poisoning.

What is the most important prognostic indicator of a poor outcome?

A aspartate transaminase

B serum urea

C alanine transferase

D serum alkaline phosphatase

E pH

## Question 3

A 19-year-old male was brought to Casualty on a cold winter's day, the day after a New Year's Eve party, by an undercover policeman, having been found collapsed on the street. They had phoned his employers, who confirmed that he had been totally well at work five hours previously and in fact had been looking forward to getting married soon. No other history was available. On examination, he was cyanosed, he had a temperature of 41.8°C, and was generally floppy except around his mouth, where he seemed to be chewing. His pulse was sinus rhythm with a rate of 165/min, and his blood pressure 80/68 mmHg. He had fixed dilated pupils. There was no neck stiffness or papilloedema and no focal neurological signs were elicited.

**Blood tests:**

| | |
|---|---|
| serum sodium | 140 mmol/L |
| serum potassium | 4.4 mmol/L |
| serum urea | 5.5 mmol/L |
| haemoglobin | 13 g/L |
| lumbar puncture | normal |

What is the most likely diagnosis?

A infection

B neuroleptic malignant syndrome

C heatstroke

D 'ecstasy' abuse (abuse of 3,4-methylenemethamphematine [MDMA])

E Addisonian crisis

## Question 4

A 23-year-old lady, whose father suffers from epilepsy, presents with nystagmus, slurred speech and ataxia. Her father is extremely distressed, and can only recall that she has been becoming progressively more drowsy within the last 24 hours. Her MRI scan on admission to hospital is normal.

The most likely diagnosis is:

A von Hippel-Lindau disease

B phenytoin toxicity

C cerebellar glioma

D acute cerebellar haemorrhage

E alcoholic cerebellar degeneration

## Question 5

A 19-year-old-girl was found by her father semi-conscious in her bedroom. She was surrounded by empty packets of his medication, which consisted of digoxin and aspirin. There was also evidence that she may have co-ingested a large amount of alcohol. She was last seen eight hours previously and her father estimated that she could have taken the tablets at any time since then. On arrival to hospital she had a Glasgow Coma Scale of 13, a pulse rate of 40 beats per minute and blood pressure 80/50 mmHg. A 12-lead ECG showed a bradycardia of 38 beats per minute with a 2:1 heart block. Initial investigations are given below. She had a good initial response with intravenous atropine, which transiently increased her heart rate to 60 beats per minute but her blood pressure remained low at < 90 mmHg systolic. However, shortly after the intravenous atropine she started having intermittent episodes of broad complex tachycardia.

| | |
|---|---|
| serum sodium | 140 mmol/L |
| serum potassium | 5.9 mmol/L |
| serum chloride | 98 mmol/L |
| serum bicarbonate | 20 mmol/L |
| serum urea | 9.2 mmol/L |
| serum creatinine | 130 µmol/L |
| plasma glucose | 5.2 mmol/L |
| digoxin level | 8 nmol/L |
| salicylate level | < 10 mg/dL |
| arterial blood gases | normal |
| full count | normal |

What would be the most appropriate treatment for this patient?

**A** bicarbonate infusion

**B** digibind (digoxin specific antibodies)

**C** haemodialysis

**D** temporary pacing wire

**E** insulin and dextrose infusion

## Question 6

A 42-year-old homeless man is brought into the Accident and Emergency Department at approximately 11pm by the emergency ambulance crew. He is known to have a history of alcohol abuse and on this occasion he was found by a group of passers-by outside a nightclub, having sustained a laceration to his forehead following a fall onto the pavement. On arrival to Accident and Emergency Department, he was described as being unkempt with a strong odour of alcohol. He was complaining of abdominal pain, nausea and blurred vision. He appeared to be moderately intoxicated with alcohol and, on examination, he was found to have a superficial laceration over his left forehead, which required no suturing. His Glasgow Coma Scale was 14, he had dilated pupils bilaterally and he had evidence of mild bilateral optic atrophy. On examination of the central nervous system no localising signs were found. He was admitted overnight for observations. He took his own discharge at approximately 9 a.m. the next day but returned to the ward later on the same day complaining of shortness of breath and blurred vision. In addition, he had developed abdominal pain associated with vomiting and diarrhoea. On examination, he had a respiratory rate of 30/min, pulse rate of 100/min regular, blood pressure of 110/60 mmHg and normal heart sounds. There were occasional coarse crepitations in both lung fields which cleared on coughing. Examination of the abdomen revealed generalised tenderness with no masses or hepatosplenomegaly. Rectal examination was normal. The only other positive findings were hyperaemia and blurring of the optic discs bilaterally.

**Initial investigations revealed:**

**Blood tests:**

| | |
|---|---|
| bicarbonate | 16 mmol/L |
| base excess | –12 |
| serum sodium | 128 mmol/L |
| serum potassium | 4.1 mmol/L |
| serum urea | 7.2 mmol/L |
| serum creatinine | 113 µmol/L |
| serum chloride | 106 mmol/L |
| plasma glucose | 11.4 mmol/L |
| serum amylase | 72 iU/L |

**Arterial gases, on air:**

| | |
|---|---|
| pH | 7.25 |
| $pO_2$ | 14.3 kPa |
| $pCO_2$ | 3.7 kPa |

What is the most likely explanation?

A diabetic ketoacidosis

B ethanol overdose

C ethylene glycol ingestion

D methanol ingestion

E acute pancreatitis

## Question 7

A 23-year-old advertising trainee is brought into the Casualty department one December morning by her boyfriend, in a drowsy state. The patient lives alone in a one bedroom flat. She is normally fit and well although had recently been complaining of difficulty concentrating in lectures. She smokes 20 cigarettes a day. She was on no medication and had no previous medical history of note. She had vomited. On examination she was flushed. She had a bounding pulse of 120/min. Her blood pressure was 180/100 mmHg. Oxygen saturations were normal.

**Initial investigations revealed:**

| **Blood tests:** | |
|---|---|
| haemoglobin | 12.8 g/L |
| white cell count | $10.5 \times 10^9$/L |
| platelet count | $280 \times 10^9$/L |
| serum sodium | 134 mmol/L |
| serum potassium | 3.6 mmol/L |
| serum urea | 7.4 mmol/L |
| serum creatinine | 80 μmol/L |
| drug toxicology screen | negative |

**Further tests:**
**Arterial blood gases, on air:**

| | |
|---|---|
| $pO_2$ | 8.6 kPa |
| $pCO_2$ | 4.7 kPa |
| pH | 7.42 |

| | |
|---|---|
| **Chest x-ray:** | normal |

Which investigation should confirm the diagnosis?

A blood glucose

B blood lactate

C carboxyhaemoglobin level

D electroencephalogram

E lumbar puncture

## Question 8

A 20-year-old man, with a known history of severe depression, is admitted semi-conscious to Casualty from an inpatient psychiatric unit. An empty bottle of pills was found in his room. Nursing observations stated that he was mildly hypertensive, and that his pupils were equal and dilated and responded sluggishly to light. Neurological screen demonstrated global hyperreflexia. ECG demonstrated a broad-complex tachycardia.

How would you treat this patient?

A DC cardioversion

B intravenous amiodarone

C intravenous magnesium sulphate

D intravenous sodium bicarbonate

E oral activated charcoal

## Question 9

A 45-year-old, who has been suffering from schizophrenia for just over twenty-nine years, is admitted to hospital for investigation of painless jaundice. Four weeks previously he had returned from a holiday in the south of Spain. There was no history of alcohol abuse.

**Investigations revealed:**

**Blood tests:**

| | |
|---|---|
| serum sodium | 130 mmol/L |
| serum potassium | 4.1 mmol/L |
| serum urea | 4.6 mmol/L |
| serum total bilirubin | 75 µmol/L |
| serum aspartate transaminase | 67 U/L |
| serum alkaline phosphatase | 692 U/L |
| serum albumin | 39 g/L |
| serum total protein | 64 g/L |
| haematology and clotting | normal |
| abdominal ultrasound | normal |

The most likely diagnosis is:

A leptospirosis

B phenothiazine-induced cholestatic jaundice

C hepatitis A

D chronic active autoimmune hepatitis

E hepatitis C

## Question 10

A patient on long-term medication for epilepsy, had a fall and was seen in hospital with backache.

**Blood tests:**

| | |
|---|---|
| haemoglobin | 10 g/L |
| white cell count | $5 \times 10^9$/L |
| platelet count | $300 \times 10^9$/L |
| MCV | 102 fL |
| serum calcium | 1.9 mmol/L |
| serum phosphate | 0.7 mmol/L |
| serum alkaline phosphatase | 241 U/L |
| serum albumin | 32 g/L |

What is the most likely cause of her abnormal blood results?

A coeliac disease

B phenytoin therapy

C hypothyroidism

D chronic renal failure

E autoimmune hypothyroidism and hypoparathyroidism

## Question 11

A 55-year-old lady presents to Casualty with a two week history of increasing unsteadiness. She is ataxic and has bilateral nystagmus. She drinks one glass of sherry per evening and stopped smoking two years ago. Her medical history is extensive and includes peripheral vascular disease, COPD with cor pulmonale, osteoarthritis, type 2 diabetes and bipolar affective disorder. She has not brought her medication into clinic, but her son reports that she is on regular nebulisers, a long list of tablets for her diabetes, her joints and her nerves. She remembers that her GP recently started her on a water tablet for increasing fluid retention.

The most likely explanation is:

A lateral medullary syndrome

B hypercapnoea

C lithium toxicity

D uraemic encephalopathy

E alcohol

## Question 12

A 65-year-old lady with a 6 year history of rheumatoid arthritis treated with intramuscular gold injections for three months is seen in clinic. On examination, she has an active synovitis affecting the small hand joints, both wrists and the knees. Generalised soft lymphadenopathy is noted. Examination is otherwise normal. Investigations show: serum haemoglobin level 7.3 g/L, MCV 78 fL, white cell count 2.3 × $10^9$/L, platelet count 95 × $10^9$/L. Serum sodium 135 mmol/L, serum potassium 4 mmol/L, serum urea 5 mmols/L, serum albumin 40 g/L, serum total protein 53 g/L.

What is the most likely diagnosis?

A folate deficiency secondary to methotrexate

B iron deficiency secondary to NSAID use

C autoimmune pancytopaenia

D gold-induced bone marrow aplasia

E Felty's syndrome

## Question 13

A 16-year-old boy presented with a three week history of malaise, fever, cough, and progressive shortness of breath. Past medical history was unremarkable, apart from acne vulgaris for which he had been receiving antibiotics from his GP. Investigations showed: haemoglobin 12.3 g/L, white cell count 9 × $10^9$/L (50% polymorphic neutrophils, 20% lymphocytes), platelet count 230 × $10^9$/L, C-reactive protein 45 g/L, and erythrocyte sedimentation rate 57 mm in the first hour (Westergren). Serum urea and electrolytes are normal.

What is the most likely diagnosis?

A *Mycoplasma pneumoniae*

B *Legionella pneumoniae*

C Wegener's granulomatosis

D tetracycline-induced pulmonary eosinophilia

E asthma

## Question 14

A 15-year-old boy developed tonsillitis, which was treated with penicillin. However, the drug was stopped after four days because he developed diarrhoea. Five months later, he presented with bloody diarrhoea. A subsequent flexible sigmoidoscopy revealed erythematous mucosa and rectal biopsy confirmed changes consistent with ulcerative colitis. He was commenced on prednisolone and sulphasalazine, but one month later was admitted with fever, malaise and a painful mouth. On examination, he appeared unwell. His temperature was 39°C. His tongue was coated and covered with several painful ulcers. Examination of the neck revealed tender lymphadenopathy. Examination of all other systems was normal. Investigations were as follows:

| **Blood tests:** | |
|---|---|
| haemoglobin | 12 g/L |
| white cell count | 1.9 × $10^9$/L (neutrophils 0.2, lymphocytes 1.6) |
| platelet count | 110 × $10^9$/L |
| serum sodium | 135 mmol/L |
| serum potassium | 3.7 mmol/L |
| serum urea | 6 mmol/L |
| serum creatinine | 80 μmol/L |
| **Further haematology:** | Coomb's test, negative |
| **Chest x-ray:** | normal heart size, clear lung fields |

What is the underlying cause of his presentation?

A ulcerative colitis

B penicillin therapy

C sulphasalazine therapy

D prednisolone

E inherited complement deficiency

## Question 15

A 70-year-old lady with primary biliary cirrhosis and ischaemic heart disease was seen in clinic and commenced on simvastatin for a high serum cholesterol. Six weeks later, she was admitted with aches and pains all over her limbs, and had general malaise.

**Investigations revealed:**

| **Blood tests:** | |
|---|---|
| haemoglobin | 11 g/L |
| white cell count | $10 \times 10^9$/L |
| platelet count | $125 \times 10^9$/L |
| serum sodium | 131 mmol/L |
| serum potassium | 5.4 mmol/L |
| serum urea | 10 mmol/L |
| serum creatinine | 72 µmol/L |
| serum aspartate transaminase | 90 U/L |
| serum alkaline phosphatase | 546 U/L |
| serum creatine kinase | 1700 U/L |
| **ECG:** | non-specific ST segment changes in the lateral leads. |

What is the diagnosis?

A polymyositis

B osteomalacia

C polymyalgia rheumatica

D simvastatin-induced myositis

E non-ST elevation myocardial infarction

## Question 16

A 68-year-old male is referred to the Accident and Emergency Department with worsening breathlessness. This has deteriorated over the last two weeks and he has also noticed leg swelling and discomfort. He has a past history of ischaemic heart disease with congestive cardiac failure, gastro-oesophageal reflux and gout. He takes omeprazole 20 mg daily, allopurinol 100 mg daily, atorvastatin 10 mg daily, digoxin 125 mcg daily, furosemide 80 mg daily, spironolactone 10 mg daily, carvedilol 2.5 mg twice daily, ramipril 10 mg daily and has recently commenced trimethoprim 200 mg twice daily for a urinary tract infection. Examination reveals him to be slightly breathless at rest, with a blood pressure of 108/80 mmHg. His jugular venous pressure is elevated and he has peripheral oedema up to his knees. Auscultation of the heart reveals a soft systolic murmur at the apex and he has bilateral basal crepitations in his chest.

**Investigations revealed:**

**Blood tests:**

| | |
|---|---|
| serum sodium | 131 mmol/L |
| serum potassium | 4.0 mmol/L |
| serum urea | 26.5 mmol/L |
| serum creatinine | 400 µmol/L |
| plasma glucose | 5.9 mmol/L |

Which drug does not require dose reduction due to his renal impairment?

A allopurinol

B digoxin

C omeprazole

D spironolactone

E trimethoprim

## Question 17

A 72-year-old male is being treated for hypertension, gout, gastro-oesophageal reflux disease, and has a three year history of type 2 diabetes mellitus. He takes a variety of medications. His GP is concerned after requesting serum biochemistry on this patient.

**These investigations have revealed:**

**Blood tests:**

| | |
|---|---|
| serum sodium | 138 mmol/L |
| serum potassium | 4.4 mmol/L |
| serum urea | 12.8 mmol/L |
| serum creatinine | 162 μmol/L |

Of the following drugs that he takes, which one does not require dose reduction?

A allopurinol

B gliclazide

C lansoprazole

D lisinopril

E metformin

## Question 18

A 26-year-old female, on no medication, presents with three elevated blood pressure readings, 150/85, 155/90, 150/80.

What is the most likely diagnosis?

A essential hypertension

B Cushing's syndrome

C Conn's syndrome

D phaeochromocytoma

E renal artery stenosis

## Question 19

An otherwise well 63-year-old woman with hypertension is referred to an Outpatient clinic for an assessment. Despite treatment with a thiazide diuretic, a beta-adrenergic antagonist (beta-blocker) and an angiotensin converting enzyme (ACE) inhibitor her blood pressure is 178/96. Investigations show serum sodium concentration 139 mmol/L, serum potassium concentration 3.1 mmol/L, serum creatinine concentration 108 µmol/L.

What is the most likely cause of the hypokalaemia?

A a low dietary potassium intake

B excessive secretion of aldosterone

C ACE inhibitor

D beta-adrenergic antagonist

E thiazide diuretic

## Question 20

A 48-year-old female presents to you after being found to have a high blood pressure in the Well Woman Clinic. She has been generally well except for previous laparoscopic cholecystectomy for gallstones. She takes no medication and is a non-smoker. Examination reveals an obese female with a body mass index of 32.2 $kg/m^2$. The mean of three separate blood pressure measurements is 172/98 mmHg. Cardiovascular and fundal examinations are otherwise normal. Her ECG reveals no specific abnormalities.

What is the most appropriate treatment for this particular patient's blood pressure?

A ACE inhibitor

B atenolol

C calcium channel antagonist

D thiazide diuretic

E weight loss

## Question 21

A 42-year-old female, with a recent diagnosis of systemic sclerosis, is referred to hospital with a complaint of headaches and blurred vision. She has a past medical history of asthma. On examination, her blood pressure is 230/120, and there is bilateral papilloedema.

Which of the following medications should be prescribed immediately?

A intravenous furosemide

B intravenous labetalol

C intravenous sodium nitroprusside

D oral enalapril

E sublingual nifedipine

## Question 22

A 26-year-old female who is 13 weeks pregnant is seen in the Outpatient clinic and noted to have a sustained blood pressure of 170/92 mmHg. She has no past medical history of note and has otherwise been well and asymptomatic. This is her first pregnancy. Examination is otherwise normal and no abnormalities are noted on fundoscopy. Ultrasound examination of the kidneys showed both kidneys to be of equal size 9–10 cm. Urinalysis reveals protein (+) and blood (+).

What is the most appropriate anti-hypertensive therapy for this patient?

A ACE inhibitor

B alpha-methyldopa

C beta-blocker

D hydralazine

E labetalol

# Answers to Chapter 6: Clinical pharmacology and toxicology

These solutions aim to provide the reason(s) for the right answer, and also the reason(s) for the wrong answers being excluded.

1 **Answer C:** This patient has a number of possible causes of electrolyte disturbance. Dehydration from the diarrhoea alone may account for some symptoms. However, you are told that she is receiving treatment for bipolar disorder and this might consist of lithium therapy. Lithium toxicity can cause diarrhoea, but may also be precipitated by dehydration. All of the symptoms may be due to lithium toxicity (diarrhoea, tremor and dysarthria). Lithium levels should be taken, but may be of limited value in the acute setting (rapid result may not be available; levels not always reliable especially with sustained release preparations). Toxic levels of lithium occur at > 2.0 mmol/L; the therapeutic range is 0.6–1.2 mmol/L. The management of lithium toxicity is largely supportive. The first step is to establish renal function and correct serum electrolytes. Renal function will determine the patient's ability to excrete lithium. Various treatment options exist for lithium toxicity, including haemodialysis and gut decontamination.

2 **Answer E:** The three most prognostic indicators are pH, serum creatinine and international normalised ratio. Therefore, E is the only correct answer out of the options given.

3 **Answer D:** There are very few reasons for a young man to suddenly become unconscious, shocked, and hyperpyrexial with fixed pupils. The temperature is too high for a normal bacterial infection, and he is unlikely to be shocked if he has a viral infection. The most likely acute insult in this case is substance abuse and the picture is typical of the severe effects of 'ecstasy' (E, MDMA). No other substance is likely to cause this syndrome. Neuroleptic malignant syndrome is associated with muscle stiffness and there is no history of psychiatric illness. (*See* **Learning point**.)

4 **Answer B:** The clue is obvious for those in the know (!) in the second set of four words of the first sentence of the question. Her symptoms are all side effects of phenytoin toxicity.

5 **Answer B:** Clinical features of severe digoxin poisoning include hyperkalaemia, metabolic acidosis, both brady- and tachyarrythmia. Hypotension can occur due to the bradyarrhythmias and decreased cardiac contractility. Digoxin level is useful but not an absolute guide to toxicity. In absence of digoxin specific antibodies, insertion of a temporary pacing wire may improve the heart rate, but can lower the fibrillatory potential of the heart muscle and induce arrhythmias. Intravenous magnesium may be a useful temporary

antiarrhythmic agent until digibind fragments are available. (*See* **Learning point**.)

6 **Answer D:** The most obvious abnormality is a metabolic acidosis with respiratory compensation. He also has a large anion gap of 29.1, {anion gap = (Na + K)–(Chloride + HCO3), normally 12±2} which indicates the presence of a large concentration of cations. Possible diagnosis includes ethylene glycol or methanol ingestion and diabetic ketoacidosis. Ethanol can also cause an elevated anion gap. The absence of a significantly elevated glucose makes diabetic ketoacidosis potentially unlikely, although DKA can also be associated with raised anion gap even without significant hyperglycaemia. Visual impairment typically occurs with methanol and in severe cases results in permanent blindness. Initial presentation of methanol or ethylene glycol mimics those of ethanol ingestion and when co-ingested, protects the patient from the toxic effects of methanol and ethylene glycol (possibly delaying the diagnosis). This is due to alcohol dehydrogenase having a higher affinity for ethanol hence methanol and ethylene glycol are excreted unchanged in the kidneys; preventing the formation of toxic metabolites formate (methanol) and oxalic acid (ethylene glycol). Severe pancreatitis can give rise to a lactic acidosis but does not give rise to hyperaemia or blurring of the optic discs. Intravenous fomepizole is the specific treatment required immediately for this condition. Intravenous ethanol is still a recommended treatment for ethylene glycol and methanol treatment. Dialysis may be required if the patient remains acidotic.

7 **Answer C:** Drug overdose is the most common cause of unconsciousness in young people, but other diagnoses must always be considered. Carboxyhaemoglobin levels should be measured in patients found unconscious indoors or in vehicles and after known exposure to smoke. This girl has classical features of carbon monoxide poisoning. Carbon monoxide binds with haemoglobin with a greater affinity than oxygen, displacing it from the blood and causing tissue hypoxia. In addition carbon monoxide shifts the oxygen dissociation curve to the left, reducing tissue delivery even more. Symptoms of mild poisoning (carboxyhaemoglobin levels = 10–30%) are headache, tiredness, nausea, dizziness and poor concentration. With increasing levels vomiting and weakness then impaired consciousness may occur with hypertension, tachycardia and flushing. With severe poisoning (carboxyhaemoglobin levels > 50%) convulsions, coma, respiratory depression and death can occur. Papilloedema can occur in severe carbon monoxide poisoning and can account for the swollen appearance of the optic disks on fundoscopy. Treatment is with 100% hyperbaric oxygen through a tight fitting, non-rebreathing face mask at a flow rate of 10 L/min. Hyperbaric oxygen (2½ atm pressure) will decrease the elimination half-life of CO from four hours to 22 minutes, but this is not often available on-site and hence patient transfer to

a specialist centre will be required. In severe cases intubation and mechanical ventilation may be required and in these patients there is a place for hyperbaric oxygen.

8 **Answer D:** The history is suggestive of a tricyclic antidepressant (TCA) overdose. Hypertension results from the blockade of noradrenaline reuptake and is usually mild and best left untreated. Alkalinisation, activated charcoal, and sodium loading are effective in the treatment of TCA-induced conduction deficits, including ventricular arrhythmias. Prolonged QT interval on the ECG may predispose to ventricular arrhythmias. Intravenous bicarbonate may reduce the risk of arrhythmias and seizures in these situations.

9 **Answer B:** The blood results indicate a drug-induced cholestatic picture. Drugs that do this include erythromycin, rifampicin, griseofulvin, carbimazole, glibenclamide, chlorpromazine, phenobarbitotone, prochlorperazine, and thioridazine.

10 **Answer B:** Phenytoin therapy is a cause of osteomalacia, which accounts for the backache. Other possibilities include malnutrition or malabsorption. Other side-effects of phenytoin include neurological symptoms, such as confusion, ataxia and acute diplopia. Other associated side effects are the Stevens-Johnson syndrome, hirsutism, gum hypertrophy and aplastic anaemia. Coeliac disease can also cause macrocytic anaemia and osteomalacia secondary to malabsorption.

11 **Answer C:** Lithium toxicity is associated with the above: including ataxia, confusion, nystagmus and tremor.

12 **Answer D:** Gold is the most likely offending drug, and in this context may cause bone marrow aplasia.

13 **Answer D:** The big part of the differential unaccounted for is the eosinophilia. Tetracycline can cause an increased eosinophil count.

14 **Answer C:** The picture is of sulphasalazine-induced neutropenia. The management should include barrier nursing, high dose penicillin and gentamicin, intravenous aciclovir, stopping the offending drug sulphasalazine, and to perform a septic screen. The patient here presents with a high fever and sore mouth after commencing sulphasalazine for ulcerative colitis. The main clue for the right answer is in the full blood count, which reveals a neutropaenia. Sulphasalazine-induced neutropaenia is well recognised but fortunately affects a very small proportion of patients. Neutropenia predisposes to bacterial, viral and fungal infections. (*See* **Learning point**.)

15 **Answer D:** Rhabdomyolysis secondary to simvastatin treatment. This can occur particularly if it is prescribed in liver disease, in conjunction with fibrates and nicotinic acid, and if it is prescribed together with ciclosporin.

It is interesting to note that there are interactions of foods and drugs on the cytochrome P450 system, increasing the risk of rhabdomyolysis; there have also been warnings about the interactions between simvastatin and citrus flavanoids such as in grapefruit juice.

16 **Answer C:** Omeprazole is principally dependent upon hepatic clearance and is safe even with marked renal impairment. Spironolactone should probably be avoided with this degree of renal impairment, owing to the risk of hyperkalaemia. Allopurinol toxicity is increased in moderate to severe renal impairment. Although reduction in dose for trimethoprim is advocated in renal impairment, there are seldom any significant problems at a full dose. Trimethoprim is a cause of elevated serum creatinine concentrations due to impairing serum creatinine secretion.

17 **Answer C:** Allopurinol is useful in renal impairment, but the dose should be reduced from 300 mg/day to 100 mg/day in moderate to severe renal impairment, as toxicity may occur, leading to hypersensitivity rashes or hepatitis. Gliclazide dosage should be reduced in mild renal failure, and should be stopped in severe renal disease. Lansoprazole is safe to use in renal impairment (caution in liver impairment), at a dose of 15–30 mg/day. Lisinopril should be used with caution in renal impairment. It may potentiate hyperkalaemia and hypotension; therefore, the dose should be reduced to 10–20 mg/day, rather than 20–40 mg/day. Metformin excretion is impaired in renal failure, subsequently predisposing lactic acidosis and therefore should be reduced with mild renal impairment. General advice suggests stopping with an eGFR < 30.

18 **Answer A:** Two forms of high blood pressure have been described: essential (or primary) hypertension and secondary hypertension. Essential hypertension is a far more common condition and accounts for 95% of hypertension. The cause of essential hypertension is multifactorial: that is, there are several factors whose combined effects produce hypertension. In secondary hypertension, which accounts for 5% of hypertension, the high blood pressure is secondary to (caused by) a specific abnormality in one of the organs or systems of the body. Even in this age group, essential hypertension is the most likely diagnosis.

19 **Answer E:** Treatment with thiazides causes mild hypokalaemia, owing to increased sodium reabsorption and hence increased potassium secretion in the distal convoluted tubules of the kidneys. Excessive secretion of aldosterone (Conn's syndrome) causes hypokalaemia and hypertension, but is an uncommon cause of hypertension. Hypokalaemia is rarely due to a low dietary potassium intake alone. ACE inhibitors cause mild (usually) hyperkalaemia.

20 **Answer E:** This obese patient has confirmed hypertension, which is associated with no evidence of target organ damage. Consequently, the most

appropriate intervention to improve blood pressure control would be weight loss. Studies indicate that a weight loss of 5 kg is associated with as much as a 10 mmHg of systolic blood pressure. Similarly, advocating a low salt diet, restricting alcohol consumption, stopping smoking and increasing exercise are all important manoeuvres. The British Hypertension Society guidelines recommend three months of lifestyle intervention and if this does not succeed in achieving adequate BP control then drug therapy is required.

21 **Answer D:** This is a relatively favourite topic of the MRCP Parts 1 and 2 Written Examination. Systemic sclerosis is a systemic disorder characterised by skin thickening due to the deposition of collagen in the dermis. Adverse prognostic features are renal, cardiac or pulmonary involvement. A major complication is the development of scleroderma renal crisis. This is characterised by the abrupt onset of severe hypertension (abrupt onset), usually with grade III or IV retinopathy, together with rapid deterioration of renal function and heart failure; haematological tests often demonstrate a thrombocytopaenia and/or microangiopathic haemolysis. It develops in 8–15% of patients with diffuse systemic sclerosis, especially associated with rapid progression of diffuse skin disease. It usually presents early, within three years of diagnosis. The pathogenic mechanisms leading to renal damage are not known. The clinical presentation is typically with the symptoms of malignant hypertension, with headaches, blurred vision, fits and heart failure. Renal function is impaired and usually deteriorates rapidly. The hypertension is almost always severe, with a diastolic BP over 100 mmHg in 90% of patients. There is hypertensive retinopathy in about 85% of patients, with exudates and haemorrhages and, if severe, papilloedema. Scleroderma renal crisis is a medical emergency. The hypertension should be treated with an ACE inhibitor. The aim is to reduce the blood pressure gradually, as an abrupt fall can lead to cerebral ischaemia or infarctions (as in any accelerated hypertension). Calcium channel blockers may be added to ACE inhibitors. Deterioration in renal function can be rapid, with gross pulmonary oedema; therefore, patients with scleroderma renal crisis should be managed in hospitals with facilities for dialysis.

22 **Answer B:** Methyldopa is the safest agent to use in the first and second trimester of pregnancy. Beta blockers may cause intrauterine growth retardation. Manufacturers recommend avoidance of hydralazine and ACE-I in pregnancy.

# Learning Points

## *Question 3*

### Learning point

**Causes of hyperpyrexia**

- Infection or septicaemia
- Malaria
- Prostaglandin therapy
- Thyroid storm
- Phaeochromocytoma
- Lithium or salicylate toxicity
- Heatstroke
- Cerebrovascular accident
- Neuroleptic malignant syndrome
- Malignant hyperthermia
- Monoamine oxidase inhibitor overdose
- Substance abuse: 'ecstasy', amphetamine, methamphetamine, cocaine

## *Question 5*

### Learning point

**Indications for digoxin-specific antibodies**

- Severe hyperkalaemia (> 6 mmol/L) resistant to treatment with insulin and dextrose (NOT calcium gluconate – risk of further ventricular arrhythmias)
- Bradyarrhythmia unresponsive to atropine with cardiac compromise (hypotension)
- Tachyarrhythmia (esp. ventricular tachycardia) associated with cardiac compromise

(Digoxin-specific antibodies should be considered at an earlier stage if the patient has pre-existing cardiac disease.)

## *Question 14*

### Learning point

**Complications secondary to sulphasalazine relatively commonly encountered in the MRCP**

- Eosinophilic syndromes (particularly pneumonitis)
- Oxidative haemolytic anaemia and methaemoglobinaemia
- Stevens-Johnson syndrome
- Hepatic granulomas
- Neutropaenia
- Cholestasis

**Causes of neutropaenia**

- Drugs (antithyroid, sulphonamides, anticonvulsants, NSAIDs, antibiotics such as chloramphenicol), phenothiazines, any drug used in chemotherapy
- Malignancy (lymphomas, leukaemias)
- Radiotherapy
- Infections (tuberculosis, viral infections)
- Megaloblastic anaemia
- Toxins (alcohol)

## CHAPTER 7

# Gastroenterology and hepatology

This section intends to examine knowledge of clinical nutrition, disorders of the mouth, tongue and salivary glands, disorders of oesophagus and stomach (including achalasia, carcinomas, peptic ulceration, gastritis and gastrointestinal haemorrhage), functional disorders (including irritable bowel syndrome), disorders of the small intestine, disorders of the liver, biliary tree and pancreas, the acute abdomen (including perforated viscus, intestinal obstruction and ischaemic bowel), the inflammatory bowel disorders (mainly Crohn's, ulcerative colitis, infective gastroenteritis), and colorectal disorders (including polyps, carcinoma, diverticular disease, and anorectal disorders).

# Questions

## Question 1

A 32-year-old lady in the last trimester of her pregnancy is referred to the medical registrar on call by the night shift in obstetrics nursing at 3 a.m. because of recent onset (within the previous few days) of generalised severe pruritis. She is recorded in the nursing notes as having passed dark urine, and pale stools.

**Investigations revealed:**

**Blood tests:**

| | |
|---|---|
| haemoglobin | 13.9 g/L |
| white cell count | 12.5 × $10^9$/L |
| platelet count | 310 × $10^9$/L |
| international normalised ratio | 1.1 |
| serum sodium | 141 mmol/L |
| serum potassium | 4.9 mmol/L |
| serum urea | 4.5 mmol/L |
| serum creatinine | 75 μmol/L |
| serum total bilirubin | 19 μmol/L |
| serum total protein | 65 g/L |
| serum albumin | 38 g/L |
| serum alanine aminotransferase | 150 U/L |
| serum alkaline phosphatase | 245 U/L |
| serum gamma glutamyl transferase | 90 U/L |
| serum amylase | 100 U/L |

What is the most likely diagnosis?

A progressive familial intrahepatic cholestasis

B cholestasis of pregnancy

C HELLP syndrome

D acute pancreatitis

E inborn errors of bile synthesis

## Question 2

A 56-year-old man presents with glycosuria. He is slightly overweight. His mother had non-insulin-dependent diabetes mellitus. Two years ago, he underwent a gastrectomy for a gastric carcinoma. He has been told that he should have regular vitamin injections. He is otherwise well. He undergoes a glucose-tolerance test.

| time (hours) | 0 | ½ | 1 | 1½ | 2 |
|---|---|---|---|---|---|
| plasma glucose (mmol/L) | 4.8 | 14.3 | 9.0 | 3.5 | 3.4 |

The most likely diagnosis is:

A post-gastrectomy

B liver failure

C diabetes mellitus

D impaired glucose tolerance

E normal glucose handling

## Question 3

A 55-year-old farmer presents with weight loss of 1 stone over three months, bilateral pitting oedema of the legs, ascites and alopecia totalis. He drinks three pints of beer a night and smokes 5 cigarettes per day. He is noted to be hyper-pigmented, and his nails are markedly dystrophic. JVP +1 cm, BP 160/90 mmHg with no postural drop, heart sounds normal and chest clear. Investigations showed Hb 10 g/dL, MCV 70 fL, white cell count 7 × $10^9$/L, platelet 245 × $10^9$/L. Liver function tests are normal apart from a serum albumin of 19 g/L. Serum sodium 140 mmol/L, serum potassium 4.0 mmol/L, serum urea 6 mmol/L, serum creatinine 101 mmol/L, PT 12 seconds, APTT 32 seconds, serum C-reactive protein < 8 g/dL. Urinalysis was negative.

The most likely cause of the low serum albumin is:

A nephrotic syndrome

B cirrhosis

C malnutrition

D protein-losing enteropathy

E elevated acute phase response

## Question 4

A 34-year-old man with a diagnosis of Crohn's disease is treated with steroids to induce remission.

Which of the following medications is most effective in maintaining remission in this patient?

**A** azathioprine

**B** budesonide

**C** ciclosporin

**D** methotrexate

**E** sulphasalazine

## Question 5

A 28-year-old trainee accountant presents with weight loss of one stone in four weeks, mild diarrhoea and mild abdominal pain. She had also noticed increasing tiredness for some months. She had not travelled abroad recently. Her family history revealed only that her mother was suffering from hyperthyroidism. On examination, she had a body mass index of 20 kg/m$^2$, pale with koilonychia, a reddened tongue, and an anaphthous ulcer on the soft palate. Abdominal and rectal examinations were normal.

| **Blood tests:** | |
|---|---|
| haemoglobin | 6.7 g/L |
| MCV | 70 fL |
| MCH | 29 pg |
| platelet count | 192 × 10$^9$/L |
| red cell folate | 47 μg/L |
| serum ferritin | 15 μg/L |
| serum vitamin $B_{12}$ | 323 ng/L |
| serum C-reactive protein | < 10 mg/L |
| erythrocyte sedimentation rate | 5 mm/hr (Westergren) |
| serum urea and electrolytes | normal |
| serum corrected calcium | 1.99 mmol/L |
| plasma free T4 | 14.5 pmol/L |
| plasma thyroid-stimulating hormone | 0.8 mU/L |
| serum total protein | 65 g/L |
| serum albumin | 34 g/L |
| serum total bilirubin | 15 μmol/L |
| serum alanine aminotransferase | 103 U/L |
| serum aspartate aminotransferase | 150 U/L |
| serum alkaline phosphatase | 146 U/L |
| serum gamma glutamyl transferase | 99 U/L |
| serum IgG | 15 mg/L |
| serum IgA | < 0.1 mg/L |
| serum IgM | 2.0 g/L |
| anti-endomysial IgA antibody | negative |
| **Blood film:** | dimorphic red cells |

The most likely diagnosis is:

A coeliac disease

B Crohn's disease

C ulcerative colitis

D intestinal lymphoma

E Whipple's disease

## Question 6

A 40-year-old man has a history of left-sided Crohn's colitis. Though previously treated with steroids and mesalazine, he has had several relapses in the past year. The last relapse, treated with high doses of steroids, was complicated by gastric bleeding.

| **Investigations revealed:** | |
|---|---|
| haemoglobin | 10.7 g/L |
| white cell count | $10 \times 10^9$/L |
| MCV | 76 fL |
| MCH | 24 pg |
| platelet count | $400 \times 10^9$/L |
| serum total protein | 70 g/L |
| serum albumin | 30 g/L |
| serum C-reactive protein | 30 mg/L |
| **Abdominal x-ray:** | normal |

What is the most appropriate next step in the management?

A a trial of oral metronidazole for three months

B total colectomy with ileostomy construction

C total colectomy with pouch construction

D treatment with azathioprine

E treatment with oral budesonide

## Question 7

A 14-year-old boy, of white Irish parents, is admitted with haematemesis. Gastroscopy demonstrates bleeding oesophageal varices. Despite being born prematurely at 32 weeks he has been completely well until presentation. On examination, there are no peripheral stigmata of chronic liver disease, but there is a palpable spleen 4 cm below the costal margin. Invasive venous pressures are as follows:

| | |
|---|---|
| hepatic wedge pressure | 8 mmHg (NR < 7) |
| inferior vena cava pressure | 3 mmHg (NR < 5) |

What is the most likely diagnosis?

A sarcoidosis

B longstanding portal vein thrombosis

C hepatic vein thrombosis

D schistomiasis

E alpha 1-antitrypsin deficiency

## Question 8

A 24-year-old businessman, who had recently spent two months in Thailand, was referred to clinic with the following blood results:

| | |
|---|---|
| serum total bilirubin | 8 mmol/L |
| serum alanine aminotransferase | 34 iU/L |
| HBsAg | positive |
| HBeAg | positive |
| Anti-HBe | negative |

Which of the following is true?

A HBV DNA levels will guide management

B liver biopsy at this stage is mandatory

C pre-core mutation should be excluded

D treatment is necessary as a priority

E he should be screened for HIV and hepatitis C

## Question 9

A 38-year-old man has a history of twelve years of IVDU, but no alcohol abuse. He is referred with the following results:

| | |
|---|---|
| HbsAg | negative |
| anti-HBc | positive |
| anti-HBs | positive |
| anti-HCV | positive |
| HCV genotype | 3a |
| serum alanine aminotransferase | 92 U/L |
| serum total bilirubin | 8 µmol/L |

Which of the following is an appropriate evidence-based statement?

A he has a 30% chance of having cirrhosis on liver biopsy

B he should receive hepatitis B vaccination

C he has a 15–20% chance of infecting a sexual partner if not using barrier contraception

D he has > 70% chance of clearing HCV with antiviral therapy

E he has a 4% per year risk of developing hepatoma

## Question 10

A 26-year-old architect (who had just finished his six-year degree) in Hampstead in London, who cooked out of iron and copper thali pots, presented to his local GP with problems in his handwriting, which had always been neat and tidy since childhood. His girlfriend had noticed that he had become increasingly irritable at home, and, against a background of general intellectual deterioration, was particularly noticed to be perseverating on the detail of one of his projects seemingly unnecessarily. His only complaint was of excessive salivation. His previous medical history was unremarkable, apart from a hernia repair as an infant. He drank about three glasses of wine a day in the evening, and was a lifelong non-smoker. His father was thought to suffer from Parkinson's disease. Examination revealed a unilateral resting tremor, with bradykinesia of the upper limbs.

**Investigations revealed:**

**Blood tests:**

| | |
|---|---|
| serum sodium | 134 mmol/L |
| serum potassium | 14.2 mmol/L |
| serum urea | 8.2 mmol/L |
| serum creatinine | 103 µmol/L |
| haemoglobin | 13 g/L |
| white cell count | 5 × $10^9$/L (normal differential count) |
| serum total bilirubin | 70 µmol/L |
| serum alanine aminotransferase | 160 U/L |
| serum aspartate transferase | 360 U/L |
| serum albumin | 35 g/L |

**Immunoglobulins:**

| | |
|---|---|
| serum IgG | 18 g/L |
| serum IgA | 3.2 g/L |
| serum IgM | 32.1 g/L |
| HbsAg, HbeAg | negative |
| anti-mitochrondrial antibodies | negative |
| serum caeruloplasmin | 0.04 g/L |
| total serum copper | 5 µmol/L (NR 11–22 µmol/L) |

**Further tests:**

| | |
|---|---|
| 24-hour urinary copper collection | 1.2 mg/a day (NR 0.01–0.06 mg/day) |

The most likely diagnosis is:

A alcoholic liver disease

B primary biliary cirrhosis

C prolonged biliary obstruction

D acaeruloplasminaemia

E Wilson's disease

## Question 11

A 30-year-old postgraduate student from China complained of generalised malaise (all the time), but was not on medication. She found herself unable to sleep at night but was drowsy during the day.

**Investigations revealed:**

| | |
|---|---|
| serum sodium | 134 mmol/L |
| serum potassium | 4.2 mmol/L |
| serum urea | 8.2 mmol/L |
| serum creatinine | 103 µmol/L |
| haemoglobin | 13 g/L |
| white cell count | $5 \times 10^9$/L (normal differential count) |
| serum total bilirubin | 70 µmol/L |
| serum alanine aminotransferase | 160 U/L |
| serum aspartate transferase | 360 U/L |
| serum albumin | 35 g/L |

**Immunoglobulins:**

| | |
|---|---|
| serum IgG | 24 g/L |
| serum IgA | 4 g/L |
| serum IgM | 3.8 g/L |
| HbsAg, HbeAg | negative |
| serology for infectious mononucleosis | negative |
| rubella and measles antibodies | high titres |
| ANA | 1/1280, diffuse homogeneous |
| anti-SMA antibodies | 1/640 |
| anti-mitochrondrial antibodies | antibodies positive |

The most likely diagnosis is:

A hepatitis A

B hepatitis B

C hepatitis C

D chronic active autoimmune hepatitis (CAH)

E rubella

## Question 12

A 56-year-old female is referred by her GP, who notes hepatomegaly. She was diagnosed with diabetes mellitus around five years previously, and takes metformin 500 mg tds and gliclazide 80 mg. She stopped smoking at the age of thirty. She drinks around 10 units of ethanol per week. On examination, she had a BMI of 37 kg/m$^2$. There were no stigmata of chronic liver disease, but there was 6 cm hepatomegaly below the costal margin.

| **Blood tests:** | |
|---|---|
| serum sodium | 134 mmol/L |
| serum potassium | 4.2 mmol/L |
| serum urea | 8.2 mmol/L |
| serum creatinine | 103 µmol/L |
| haemoglobin | 13 g/L |
| white cell count | 5 × 10$^9$/L (normal differential count) |
| serum total bilirubin | 11 µmol/L |
| serum alanine aminotransferase | 150 U/L |
| serum aspartate transferase | 100 U/L |
| serum albumin | 40 g/L |
| serum ferritin | 434 mg/L |
| **Immunoglobulins:** | |
| serum IgG | 14 g/L |
| serum IgA | 3 g/L |
| serum IgM | 2.2 g/L |
| ANA titre | negative |
| HbsAg, HbeAg | negative |
| **Ultrasound of the abdomen:** | bright echogenic liver, with gallstones noted in the gallbladder |

The most likely diagnosis is:

A alcoholic liver disease

B non-alcoholic fatty liver disease (NAFLD)

C drug-induced hepatitis

D gallstone disease

E haemochromatosis

## Question 13

A 47-year-old businessman presented to General Medical Outpatients following referral by his GP.

**Investigations revealed:**

| | |
|---|---|
| serum sodium | 134 mmol/L |
| serum potassium | 4.2 mmol/L |
| serum urea | 8.2 mmol/L |
| serum creatinine | 103 µmol/L |
| haemoglobin | 13 g/L (normal differential count) |
| white cell count | 5 × $10^9$/L |
| serum total bilirubin | 11 µmol/L |
| serum ferritin | 592 mg/L |
| serum iron | 29 µmol/L |
| serum iron binding capacity | 46 µmol/L |
| iron saturation | 63% |

**Immunoglobulins:**

| | |
|---|---|
| serum IgG | 12 g/L |
| serum IgA | 2.3 g/L |
| serum IgM | 1.2 g/L |
| ANA titre | negative |
| HbsAg, HbeAg | negative |

He had a family history of haemochromatosis.

What is the most appropriate next step in his management?

**A** genetic testing for HFE mutations

**B** begin a venesection programme

**C** monitor his serum ferritin regularly

**D** take no action until the iron saturation > 90%

**E** undertake a liver biopsy as soon as possible

## Question 14

A 52-year-old freelancing female journalist presented with a six month of dyspnoea, weight loss and diarrhoea. Over this period of time, she had lost approximately 10 kg in weight and was aware of watery diarrhoea three to four times daily. She was also aware of occasional flushes, which she had experienced since the menopause at the age of 49, but these had become more frequent of late. She reported being occasionally wheezy and breathless. She had previously been well, with no other medical history of note. She took no medication. She was a lifelong non-smoker and drank approximately 15 units of alcohol weekly. On examination, she appeared slightly plethoric and had a BMI of 24 kg/m$^2$. She had a pulse of 88/min regular and a blood pressure of 130/80 mmHg. There were no abnormalities on cardiovascular or respiratory examination, apart from a soft systolic murmur at the left sternal edge. Abdominal examination revealed two finger breadths hepatomegaly.

**Investigations revealed:**

| **Blood tests:** | |
|---|---|
| haemoglobin | 14.5 g/L |
| white blood cells | 8.2 × 10$^9$/L |
| platelet count | 300 × 10$^9$/L |
| serum sodium | 144 mmol/L |
| serum potassium | 4.1 mmol/L |
| serum urea | 3.9 mmol/L |
| serum creatinine | 110 µmol/L |
| serum total bilirubin | 13 µmol/L |
| serum aspartate aminotransferase | 60 U/L |
| serum alkaline phosphatase | 130 U/L |
| 24-hour urinary collection of 5-HIAA | 100 mg/day |
| **Abdominal ultrasound:** | echodense deposits within the liver |
| **Echocardiogram:** | marked tricuspid regurgitation, mild pulmonary stenosis |

The most appropriate empirical treatment for this patient's diarrhoea is:

**A** cryproheptadine

**B** ketanserin

**C** loperamide

**D** methysergide

**E** ocreotide

## Question 15

A 56-year-old retired Hungarian chef presents with general lethargy, weight gain and abdominal distension. His symptoms have deteriorated gradually over the previous three months, and he confesses to longstanding alcohol abuse. Currently, he is taking no medication, and previous medical history is otherwise unremarkable. Examination reveals that he is well orientated, is apyrexial, and has a blood pressure of 130/90 mmHg. He has numerous spider naevi present on the face and upper chest, and mild gynaecomastia. Abdominal examination reveals moderate ascites, he has oedema of the legs up to the mid thigh, and small testes. No organomegaly is noted on abdominal examination.

**Investigations reveal:**

**Blood tests:**

| | |
|---|---|
| serum sodium | 139 mmol/L |
| serum potassium | 4.3 mmol/L |
| serum urea | 6.9 mmol/L |
| serum creatinine | 120 µmol/L |
| serum total bilirubin | 36 µmol/L |
| serum aspartate aminotransferase | 70 U/L |
| serum alkaline phosphatase | 230 U/L |
| serum albumin | 21 g/L |

What is the best initial management step?

A drain 4L ascitic fluid

B transcutaneous liver biopsy

C surgical shunt

D commence ACE-inhibitor

E commence spironolactone

## Question 16

A 58-year-old woman, with known alcoholic liver cirrhosis, presents with vague abdominal pains, malaise and nausea. She has been abstinent since she was diagnosed eight months ago. On examination, she had moderate ascites, and mild, generalised, abdominal tenderness.

**Investigations revealed:**

**Blood tests:**

| | |
|---|---|
| haemoglobin | 11.2 g/L |
| white cell count | $15 \times 10^9$/L |
| prothrombin time | 21 s |
| serum sodium | 139 mmol/L |
| serum potassium | 4.3 mmol/L |
| serum urea | 6.9 mmol/L |
| serum creatinine | 120 µmol/L |
| serum total bilirubin | 56 µmol/L |
| serum aspartate aminotransferase | 70 U/L |
| serum albumin | 28 g/L |

**Ascitic fluid analysis:**

| | |
|---|---|
| ascitic fluid protein | 26 g/L |
| ascitic fluid white cell count | $500 \times 10^9$/L |
| ascitic fluid amylase | normal |

What is the most likely reason for her current problem?

A hepatic vein thrombosis

B pancreatic pseudocyst rupture

C portal vein thrombosis

D hepatocellular cancer

E spontaneous bacterial peritonitis

## Question 17

A 52-year-old male administrator for a Local Research Ethics Committee presented with recurrent bouts of fever over the last six months. He had lost a kilogram in weight. He had some discomfort in the right upper abdomen when he lay on his right side. He thought that he had been jaundiced at the beginning of the illness and that his stools had been pale at that time. He had been itching for about three months. A year previously, he had dark urine and frequency of micturition. At the age of 32, he had a cholecystectomy for gallstones and at 40 an operation for 'gravel' in the bile ducts. There were no other abnormal features in his past history. He had never drunk more than ten units of alcohol per week.

On examination, he was anaemic and mildly jaundiced. His blood pressure was 130/60 mmHg and pulse 98/min and regular. The temperature was 39°C. He had moderately extensive psoriasis, a few scratch marks, and there were spider naevi on the upper trunk. He had palmar erythema and white nails. The apex beat was not displaced, the first sound was quiet, and on examination of the lungs there were a few crepitations at the left base. The spleen tip was palpable two centimetres below the costal margin. The liver was slightly tender, palpable four centimetres below the costal margin and firm but not nodular. There was no ascites. There were no other abnormal signs. The urine contained traces of serum total bilirubin and protein but no glucose; microscopy was normal.

**Investigations revealed:**

**Blood tests:**

| | |
|---|---|
| haemoglobin | 10.5 g/L |
| white blood cells | 7.8 × $10^9$/L |
| platelet count | 150 × $10^9$/L |
| MCV | 105 fL |
| international normalised ratio | 1.6 |
| serum total bilirubin | 63 µmol/L |
| serum aspartate aminotransferase | 60 U/L |
| serum alkaline phosphatase | 340 U/L |
| serum lactate dehydrogenase | 350 U/L |
| serum total protein | 62 g/L |
| serum albumin | 28 g/L |
| HBsAg | negative |

**Blood film:** mild macrocytosis and occasional target cells

The most likely cause of his symptoms in the last six months is:

A primary sclerosing cholangitis

B primary biliary cirrhosis

C cholangiocarcinoma

D recurrent cholangitis

E secondary biliary cirrhosis

# Answers to Chapter 7: Gastroenterology and hepatology

These solutions aim to provide the reason(s) for the right answer, and also the reason(s) for the wrong answers being excluded.

1 **Answer B:** The diagnosis is cholestasis of pregnancy. The goals of treating this condition are to relieve the pruritis and prevent maternal and foetal complications. Fetal monitoring tests can be used to check the well-being of the foetus. Ursodeoxycholic acid can significantly reduce pruritis. If cholestasis of pregnancy endangers the well-being of the mother or foetus, then an early delivery may be necessary. Serum gamma glutamyl transferase would be expected to be normal or low in the case of progressive familial intrahepatic cholestasis or inborn errors of bile acid synthesis. The platelet count is normal and there is no evidence of a haemolytic anaemia, thus excluding HELLP syndrome. The amylase is not sufficiently high for acute pancreatitis.

2 **Answer A:** The data demonstrate a 'lag-storage' curve, the causes for which are post-gastrectomy and liver failure. In a so-called 'lag-storage' curve, there is a 1-hour glucose peak in the 11–15 mmol/L range, which then returns to normal at two hours. This is seen when a carbohydrate load rapidly reaches the small intestine and is absorbed before insulin action has time to bring down the glucose peak.

3 **Answer D:** The diagnosis is rare, Kronkite-Canada syndrome, D, but the rest are possible and can be excluded on the basis of the normal serum C-reactive protein, normal liver function tests and clotting (to infer that the low serum albumin is not related to impaired synthetic function of the liver), and negative urinalysis. The features of this rare disorder are polyps, alopecia, pigmentation, distorted nails. The causes of a low serum albumin essentially include an increase in catabolism, or a decrease in intake.

4 **Answer A:** Of the drugs listed, azathioprine has the most clinical experience in maintaining remission. Doses of up to 2.5 mg/kg are often used and steroids may be tailed off as a result. Appropriate monitoring for side effects, in particular bone marrow suppression, is mandatory.

5 **Answer A:** This patient has a selective IgA deficiency, a known association of coeliac disease. The symptoms, iron-deficiency anaemia, hypocalcaemia, and aphthous mouth ulceration (along with normal inflammatory markers) are all features of coeliac disease. The family history of autoimmunity would also favour this diagnosis. The anti-endomysial IgA is negative because the patient is IgA deficient. Anti-tissue transglutaminase (IgG) testing should ideally be performed. Duodenal biopsies are still recommended by most at the outset,

to confirm the diagnosis, and facilitate follow-up, in particular if there is an indequate response to a gluten-free diet.

6 **Answer D:** This patient has all the hallmarks of active Crohn's colitis that is failing to settle with first-line medical therapy. The next step is a trial of azathioprine, which is used as a steroid-sparing agent. This is particularly relevant to this particular patient, as he has had serious side-effects from previous steroid treatment. Several studies have failed to establish metronidazole as a significantly effective treatment of active Crohn's colitis, unless there are septic complications, such as an abscess or a superimposed infective colitis. Given that Crohn's disease can recur following surgery, an operation should not be embarked upon without first a trial of the second-line medical therapies such as azathioprine, its metabolite 5-mercaptopurine, or infliximab.

7 **Answer B:** The normal hepatic venous pressure means that portal hypertension is not related to post sinusoidal intrinsic liver disease such as cirrhosis (caused in children by metabolic disorders such as $\alpha$1-antitrypsin deficiency) or post-hepatic venous obstruction (hepatic vein thrombosis). The obstruction must be pre-sinusoidal. Sarcoidosis is a very rare cause of pre-sinusoidal portal hypertension, particularly in white children. Schistosomiasis is the leading cause of pre-sinusoidal hypertension worldwide but is unlikely to be found in an Irish boy. Thrombosis of the portal vein is a well-recognised complication in premature neonates due to cannulation of the umbilical vein during neonatal intensive care.

8 **Answer E:** This gentleman is most likely in the process of resolving an acute hepatitis B infection (in view of Anti-HBe +ve, your HBe Ag becomes negative). An anti-HBc IgM would indicate acute infection with both eAg +ve and sAg +ve). Follow-up of serology and liver function tests in six months will clarify this. Most importantly, he should be screened for other blood-borne pathogens at this stage.

9 **Answer D:** Response to anti-viral treatment in Hepatitis C is improved if female, under 40 years of age, less severe fibrosis grade on liver biopsy, and Hepatitis C genotypes 2 and 3.

10 **Answer E:** Decreased caeruloplasmin levels are seen in a variety of diseases causing severe liver dysfunction. Increased urinary copper excretion is seen in primary biliary cirrhosis (PBC), prolonged biliary obstruction and familial intrahepatic cholestasis. The very low caeruloplasmin levels above, however, are highly suggestive of Wilson's disease. A hepatic copper concentration of greater than 250 mcg of copper per gram of dry weight is considered the gold standard. The presence of Kayser-Fleischer rings is not pathognomic, as they can be found in other conditions such as primary biliary cirrhosis.

11 **Answer D:** Autoimmune chronic active hepatitis is suggested by high titres of ANA, elevated smooth muscle antibodies with high serum γ-globulin mainly comprising IgG, and the absence of hepatitis B antigen. The association of high titres of measles and rubella antibodies is not uncommon. Anti-LKM-1 antibodies may be positive and signify a more aggressive disease. Autoimmune diseases are associated with one another, and may be associated with polyglandular autoimmune disease.

12 **Answer B:** This picture is a hepatitic picture, rather than a cholestatic picture. Serum ferritin is not sufficiently high to be considered for haemochromatosis, and is an acute phase reactant typically increased in any inflammatory process. NAFLD is very common and is typically encountered in obese patients with a raised BMI and metabolic syndrome. (Very rarely presents with jaundice unless decompenasted cirrhosis.) Echogenic bright liver suggests fatty change in the liver. Weight reduction is the mainstay of treatment. If untreated this condition can lead to steatohepatitis and cirrhosis.

13 **Answer A:** This man is likely to have hereditary haemochromatosis (HH). Homozygous mutation (C282Y mutation) of the human iron gene (HFE gene) accounts for over 80% of cases with HHC. The diagnosis is made by genetic testing. If the diagnosis is confirmed, then treatment with venesection to achieve and maintain a serum ferritin of less than 50 ug/L. A liver biopsy is not required to make the diagnosis of HH although it may be indicated for staging and prognostic reasons, if cirrhosis is suspected.

14 **Answer E:** This patient has carcinoid syndrome, as revealed by the investigations. Carcinoid is a slowly-growing neuroendocrine tumour and symptoms of diarrhoea and flushes occur as a consequence of metastasis to the liver and hence systemic release of vasoactive compounds such as serotonin and bradykinin. Serum alkaline phosphatase is often raised, and derangement of transaminases often occurs, due to carcinoid infiltration. Liver function, however, can be quite normal despite heavy hepatic infiltration. Wheeze is a typical feature as a consequence of vasoactive compounds such as serotonin and bradykinin. It is also associated with endocardial fibrosis of the right side of the heart, which may result in right heart failure. The best treatment for symptoms of carcinoid syndrome is the somatostatin analogue, ocreotide, which improves symptoms and prognosis. Other potential treatments include hepatic artery chemo-embolisation. Relative youth offers a better prognosis. Cardiac lesions are not reversible with treatment, may deteriorate with time, and frequently patients require heart valve replacement.

15 **Answer E:** Initial management of ascites with spironolactone is appropriate, and is often successful. Large volume paracentesis is a good treatment for those intolerant of diuretics or those who have diuretic-resistant ascites. Diurectic resistant ascites is an indication for liver transplantation.

16 **Answer E:** The high white cell count in the ascites makes spontaneous bacterial peritonitis (SBP) more likely than Budd-Chiari syndrome, portal vein thrombosis, hepatocellular carcinoma, or a ruptured pancreatic pseudocyst. SBP is an important cause of hepatic decompensation and must be routinely excluded in this setting.

17 **Answer D:** The history is typical of recurrent cholangitis.

# Learning Points

## *Question 8*

### Learning point

**Portal hypertension**

Portal hypertension represents an increase of the hydrostatic pressure within the portal vein or its tributaries and is defined as an increase in the pressure gradient between the portal vein and hepatic veins or inferior vena cava; a pressure gradient of 12 mmHg is regarded as clinically significant. Portal hypertension has two components: the first is due to the intrahepatic obstruction of portal flow and the second to the transmitted pressure from the inferior vena cava. Therefore, the wedged hepatic venous pressure minus inferior vena cava pressure is the corrected sinusoidal pressure or that part of the portal pressure which is due to the intrahepatic resistance to blood flow. The causes of portal hypertension can be divided into: (1) posthepatic, (2) prehepatic, and (3) intrahepatic causes. The major posthepatic causes of PH are right-sided heart failure, constrictive pericarditis and the Budd-Chiari syndrome. The prehepatic causes of PH include portal vein thrombosis and portal compression or occlusion by biliary and pancreatic neoplasms and metastases. PH may be caused by increased flow secondary to arterioportal fistula, pancreatic arteriovenous malformations, and massive splenomegaly. The most common intrahepatic cause is cirrhosis.

## CHAPTER 8

# Respiratory medicine

Respiratory medicine in the MRCP is concerned with your understanding of common respiratory clinical conditions, including pleural effusions, occupational lung disease, malignant conditions, TB, asthma, emphysema, and cystic fibrosis. An understanding of simple respiratory investigations is required (such as lung function tests and relevant imaging).

# Questions

## Question 1

Which of the following is a bad prognostic factor in sarcoidosis?

A erythema nodosum

B lupus pernio

C caucasian

D peripheral lymphadenopathy

E facial nerve palsy

## Question 2

An 18-year-old woman presents with red, tender lumps on her shins and arthralgia. Chest x-ray shows bihilar lymphadenopathy, and clear lung fields. A clinical diagnosis of sarcoidosis is made.

Which of the following is the most appropriate management plan?

A 24-hour urinary calcium collection

B follow-up appointment with chest x-ray in three months' time

C mediastinoscopy and lymph node biopsy

D skin biopsy

E thoracic CT scan

## Question 3

In which of the following have randomised trials shown that long-term oxygen therapy (LTOT) reduces mortality?

A asthma

B chronic bronchitis

C cryptogenic fibrosing alveolitis

D cystic fibrosis

E pulmonary sarcoidosis

## Question 4

A 52-year-old man is diagnosed with a mesothelioma.

Which of the following is the most likely presenting complaint?

A chest pain

B shortness of breath

C haemoptysis

D weight loss

E increased sputum production

## Question 5

Pollens of importance in the spring, as a cause of seasonal allergic rhinitis in the UK, include:

A dogstail pollen

B birch pollen

C nettle pollen

D dock pollen

E *Alternaria* pollen

## Question 6

A 50-year-old male presented with acute respiratory failure during an episode of acute pancreatitis and was thought to have developed acute respiratory distress syndrome (ARDS).

Which of the following would support a diagnosis of ARDS?

A high pulmonary capillary wedge pressure

B high protein pulmonary oedema

C hypercapnea

D increased lung compliance

E normal chest x-ray

## Question 7

A 43-year-old woman wants to quit smoking. She is on carbamazepine for her epilepsy, a steroid inhaler, and an occasional salbutamol (when required).

The best next management step is:

A counselling

B bupropion (Zyban)

C nicotine patches

D counselling and nicotine patches

E fluoxetine

## Question 8

Which of the following is a recognised feature of massive pulmonary embolism?

A reduced plasma lactate levels

B an increase in serum troponin levels

C an arterial pH less than 7.2

D haemoptysis

E normal D dimer values

## Question 9

A 64-year-old man is found to have squamous cell bronchogenic carcinoma.

Which of the following statements is true regarding surgical resection?

A a $FEV_1$ of 2L is a major contraindication to surgical resection

B hypercalcaemia makes further assessment for surgery unnecessary

C resection is precluded if a CT scan of the thorax shows enlarged mediastinal lymph nodes

D positive sputum cytology excludes the need for bronchoscopic examination of the airways

E the presence of finger clubbing indicates that liver metastases are already present

## Question 10

A 60-year-old man is admitted with community-acquired pneumonia and deteriorates over the next few hours.

Which of the following indicates a poor prognosis?

A a total white cell count of $17 \times 10^9$/L

B blood pressure of 117/70

C respiratory rate of 35/min

D rigors

E temperature of 39°C

## Question 11

A 65-year-old lady is admitted as an emergency after a choking episode. She is breathless and has a temperature of 37.8°C. She is a smoker of around 20 cigarettes a day, but has no history of previous respiratory disease; she had a stroke six months previously. She was started on oral co-amoxiclav by her GP. A chest x-ray showed a homogenous opacity at the right base with the right hilum pulled downwards.

What is the next investigation of choice?

A blood cultures

B bronchoscopy

C CT chest

D sputum culture

E ventilation/perfusion scan

## Question 12

A 19-year-old lady developed increasing breathlessness and hypoxia two days after admission with severe burns. She had no previous history of note. Her father had had a myocardial infarction at the age of 40. She was a non-smoker. On examination, she had a respiratory rate of 26 breaths per minute and a pulse rate of 110 beats per minute. On auscultation, there are crackles audible over both lung fields. A chest x-ray revealed bilateral hazy shadowing, with air bronchograms. The heart size was normal.

What is the most likely diagnosis?

**A** adult respiratory distress syndrome

**B** chemical pneumonitis

**C** left ventricular failure

**D** nosocomial pneumonia

**E** pulmonary haemorrhage

## Question 13

A 22-year-old lady was planning to emigrate to Australia and had a chest x-ray undertaken as part of her visa requirements. This demonstrated bilateral hilar lymphadenopathy but clear lung fields. She also presented with acute stiffness and swelling of the hands and ankles, and a painful rash on the legs. The erythrocyte sedimentation rate was 96 mm in the first hour. The rash was diagnosed as erythema nodosum, and the chest x-ray was suspicious of showing sarcoidosis. She was referred to the outpatients clinic. On systems review in outpatients, a two month history of arthralgia and a dry cough was elicited. She had no previous history of note but three months ago she had had unprotected sexual intercourse and took an HIV test which was negative. She had no other symptoms. She had lived in Zimbabwe until she was 16. She worked as a waitress.

Which one investigation is most likely to confirm the diagnosis?

**A** bronchoalveolar lavage

**B** high-resolution CT scan of the chest

**C** serum ACE

**D** transbronchial biopsy

**E** tuberculin test

## Question 14

A 67-year-old man presents with a two month history of persistent cough. The cough is always unproductive and there has been no haemoptysis. It never wakes him from his sleep. He has no chest pain but has noticed some mild breathlessness on exertion. He is a smoker of 20 cigarettes a day since the age of seventeen. He has lost a small amount of weight, and has a reduced appetite. He has been constipated over the last two weeks. Examination was unremarkable. He has no clubbing nor lymphadenopathy. Examining his chest, breath sounds were vesicular with no added sounds.

| **Investigations revealed:** | |
|---|---|
| haemoglobin | 13.0 g/L |
| white cell count | $10 \times 10^9$/L |
| platelet count | $165 \times 10^9$/L |
| serum sodium | 149 mmol/L |
| serum potassium | 4.4 mmol/L |
| serum urea | 9.4 mmol/L |
| serum creatinine | 110 µmol/L |
| serum corrected calcium | 3.26 mmol/L |
| **Chest x-ray:** | right hilar lympadenopathy |

What is the next best investigation?

A bone marrow biopsy

B bronchoscopy

C CT chest

D isotope bone scan

E serum ACE

## Question 15

A 35-year-old gym teacher is admitted with a two week history of fever, cough and shortness of breath. The cough has been productive of yellow-green sputum. He had a past medical history of asthma and hayfever. On examination, he appeared flushed, febrile at 38.4°C, with a rash on his back. He is tachycardic with a pulse of 120/min. Chest expansion is reduced, with bilateral basal inspiratory and expiratory coarse crackles.

| **Investigations revealed:** | | |
|---|---|---|
| haemoglobin | 12.3 g/L | |
| white cell count | $3.5 \times 10^9$/L | |
| platelet count | $353 \times 10^9$/L | |
| **Arterial gases, on air:** | $pO_2$ | 8 kPa |
| | $pCO_2$ | 4 kPa |
| **Blood film:** | agglutinated red cells | |

Which clinical sign would most support your diagnosis?

**A** erythema marginatum

**B** bullous myringitis

**C** labial herpes simplex

**D** erysipelas

**E** erythema gyratum repens

## Question 16

A 24-year-old heterosexual male presents after developing a bluish discolouration of his body, lips and nails, appearing in Casualty with breathlessness. He denies any relevant past medical history, but his notes from a different hospital state that he has been treated for HIV previously. Due to an allergy to septrin, he is treated with a combination of dapsone and trimethoprim prophylactically for a putative diagnosis of *Pneumocystis carinii* pneumonia. Examination reveals a central cyanosis and a grey complexion.

**Investigation revealed:**

| | |
|---|---|
| haemoglobin | 17.0 g/L |
| $paO_2$ | 13.0 kPa |
| $saO_2$ using an oximeter | 85% |

Which is the likely diagnosis?

A agyria

B cyanotic congenital heart disease

C haemochromatosis

D methaemoglobinaemia

E methylene blue poisoning after a surgical parathyroidectomy

## Question 17

A 68-year-old retired plumber presents with a six month history of dry nocturnal cough and increasing exertional breathlessness. The cough is unproductive and there has been no haemoptysis. He is comfortable at rest but his breathing limits him to 400 metres on the flat and he is beginning to have difficulty climbing stairs. He sleeps with four pillows. He had a myocardial infarction four years ago and has a 15 year history of hypertension. His current treatment is aspirin, atenolol, simvastatin and bendroflumethiazine (bendrofluazide). On examination, he has finger clubbing, cyanosis and looks pale. His pulse is 48 beats per minute and is regular. Blood pressure is 156/78. On examining his chest he has vesicular breath sounds with bilateral basal crackles.

**Investigations revealed:**

| | | |
|---|---|---|
| **Arterial gases, on air:** | $paO_2$ | 8.2 kPa |
| | $paCO_2$ | 5.1 kPa |
| | pH | 7.41 |
| **Pulmonary function tests:** | $FEV_1$ | 2.3 (predicted 3.0) |
| | FVC | 2.8 (predicted 3.8) |
| | $FEV_1$/FVC | 82% |
| **ECG:** | sinus bradycardia with Q waves in the anterior chest leads and left ventricular hypertrophy | |
| **Chest x-ray:** | bilateral lower zone shadowing. | |

Which one of the following investigations is most likely to establish the diagnosis?

A echocardiography

B high resolution CT of the chest

C measurement of diffusion capacity

D serum ACE

E bronchoalveolar lavage

## Question 18

A 48-year-old teacher is admitted with a two day history of increasing breathlessness and cough productive of purulent sputum. He has smoked 20 cigarettes a day since the age of eighteen. He has not been in hospital before but was recently diagnosed by his GP as having chronic obstructive pulmonary disease. He is taking an inhaled agonist on an as-required basis. On examination he is breathless at rest, alert and orientated. He is cyanosed and has a respiratory rate of 26 breaths per minute. His temperature is 37.8 C. His pulse is 100/min and blood pressure is 150/100. Auscultation of his chest reveals bilaterally reduced air entry. His chest radiograph demonstrates a normal heart size but the lung fields are hyperinflated. There is no pneumonic consolidation. Arterial blood gases on admission (on 24% oxygen) by nasal cannulae show:

| | |
|---|---|
| pH | 7.34 |
| $pO_2$ | 6.5 kPa |
| $pCO_2$ | 6.9 kPa |
| $HCO_3$ | 27 mmol/L |

He is treated with nebulised bronchodilators and his $FIO_2$ is increased to 28%. The results of arterial blood gases repeated after 30 minutes are:

| | |
|---|---|
| pH | 7.30 |
| $pO_2$ | 7.0 kPa |
| $pCO_2$ | 8.5 kPa |
| $HCO_3$ | 28 mmol/L |

What is the most appropriate management step?

A reduce $FIO_2$ to 24%

B intubation and mechanical ventilation

C non-invasive positive pressure ventilation

D intravenous hydrocortisone

E oxygen by face mask

## Question 19

A 78-year-old lady is admitted with increasing breathlessness and a cough productive of mucoid sputum on most days; she had become more breathless over the last five days. She was a smoker of 40 cigarettes per day until three months ago. She takes becotide 200 mcg bd, salmeterol 50 mg bd and salbutamol 2 puffs as required. On examination she was obese with a BMI of 32 kg/m$^2$. She was cyanosed and pale but there was no clubbing nor lymphadenopathy. She was breathless at rest with a respiratory rate of 24/min. Pulse was 110/min and blood pressure 140/80 mmHg. Her chest was hyperinflated with expiratory wheezes and she had bilateral swollen ankles. She was treated with nebulised bronchodilators, controlled oxygen therapy, oral prednisolone, antibiotics and commenced on diuretic therapy. She improved and was discharged home five days later. On review, six weeks later, investigations revealed:

**Arterial gases, on air:**

| | |
|---|---|
| $paO_2$ | 6.9 kPa |
| $paCO_2$ | 6.8 kPa |
| pH | 7.4 |

**Pulmonary function testing:**

| | | |
|---|---|---|
| $FEV_1$ | 0.9 L | (3.2 predicted) |
| FVC | 4.2 L | (4.5 predicted) |

Which **one** of the following is the primary indication for long-term domiciliary oxygen therapy in this patient?

A cor pulmonale

B inability to get out of the house

C low $FEV_1$

D low $paO_2$

E high $paCO_2$

## Question 20

A 67-year-old lady, with a history of CREST syndrome, presented with a seven month history of progressive exertional breathlessness and dry cough. She had a reduced appetite and had lost half a stone in weight. She had no previous history of note. She had worked as a hair stylist. She kept three cats and a dog at home. She lived alone but had been coping well until now. She smoked 20 cigarettes a day. On examination, she was clubbed and cyanosed. She was pale. Pulse rate was 80 beats per minute. BP was 138/80 mmHg. Heart sounds were normal. There were bilateral fine inspiratory crackles heard at the lung bases.

**Investigations revealed:**

| | | |
|---|---|---|
| $FEV_1$ | 2.8 L | (3.6 predicted) |
| FVC | 3.1 L | (4.5 predicted) |
| Diffusion capacity | 5.1 mmol/min/kPa | (NR 6.3–11.9) |

The chest x-ray showed slight increase in basal lung markings.

What is the most likely diagnosis?

A bronchiectasis

B sclerosis-associated interstitial lung disease

C left ventricular failure

D lymphangitis carcinomatosis

E sarcoidosis

## Question 21

A 65-year-old retired miner attends the outpatient department with a six month history of breathlessness on exertion, which has got worse following a recent chest infection. He has a cough productive of mucoid sputum. He smoked 20 cigarettes a day until five years ago. He keeps pigeons at home.

**Lung function tests show:**

| | *Before bronchodilator* | *After bronchodilator* | |
|---|---|---|---|
| $FEV_1$ | 0.9 | 1.0 | (NR 2.2–4.4) |
| VC | 2.1 | 2.3 | (NR 3.0–4.8) |
| TLC | 7.2 | | (NR 2.4–4.6) |
| KCO | 0.6 | | (NR 1.2–2.1) |

What is the most likely diagnosis?

**A** asthma

**B** chronic obstructive pulmonary disease

**C** coal workers' pneumoconiosis

**D** pigeon fanciers' lung

**E** extrinsic allergic alveolitis

## Question 22

A 62-year-old lady was seen in the outpatient department with a six month history of increasing breathlessness on exertion. Her exercise tolerance was limited to 80 metres on the flat and she had started to become breathless walking up the stairs in her house. She slept with four pillows and had noticed some swelling of both her ankles. She had a cough which was occasionally productive of sputum. She had given up smoking when she first noticed her dyspnoea and had a 40 pack year smoking history. She was known to have hypertension and ischaemic heart disease and had coronary artery stenting 12 months ago.

**Pulmonary function testing revealed:**

| | | |
|---|---|---|
| $FEV_1$ | 0.82 L | (1.80–3.02 predicted) |
| FVC | 1.84 L | (2.16–3.58 predicted) |
| diffusion capacity | 2.40 mmol/min/kPa | (5.91–9.65 predicted) |
| total lung capacity | 4.40 L | (4.25–6.22 predicted) |
| residual volume | 2.9 L | (1.46–2.48 predicted) |

There was a scalloping of the expiratory loop of the flow-volume curve. A 2 week trial of oral steroids excluded reversible airway pathology.

What is the most likely diagnosis?

A asthma

B chronic obstructive pulmonary disease

C cryptogenic fibrosing alveolitis

D left ventricular failure

E sarcoidosis

## Question 23

An 18-year-old non-smoker presents with increasing breathlessness over six months, a two year history of pain in the right arm, and a 1½ year history of polyuria. Clinical examination is normal.

**Investigations reveal:**

**Blood tests:**

| | |
|---|---|
| serum sodium | 148 mmol/L |
| serum potassium | 4.2 mmol/L |
| serum urea | 6 mmol/L |
| serum creatinine | 80 µmol/L |
| plasma glucose | 5.7 mmol/L |

**Chest x-ray:** interstitial fibrosis, principally upper lobe with bilateral cystic destruction

**Arterial gases, on air:**

| | |
|---|---|
| pH | 7.4 |
| $pCO_2$ | 4.1 |
| $pO_2$ | 8.1 |
| BE | +1 |

**PFTs:**
$FEV_1$/FVC = 84%
TLC: 104% predicted
KCO: 53% predicted

**Water deprivation test:**

| | *Plasma osmolality* | *Urinary osmolality* | *Weight (kg)* |
|---|---|---|---|
| 0h | 296 | 101 | 80 |
| 8h | 331 | 128 | 72 |

The most likely diagnosis is:

A histoplasmosis

B extrinsic allergic alveolitis

C usual interstitial pneumonia

D sarcoidosis

E Langerhans' cell histiocytosis

## Question 24

A 19-year-old male university student, a lifelong non-smoker, was admitted with recurrent haemoptysis and significantly increasing breathlessness on exertion over a month's period. He had remembered having these symptoms in milder form beginning roughly at the age of 3½. On admission, he was pale, dyspnoeic with an increased respiratory rate of 28 breaths/minute at rest and no fever. Ausculation of the chest revealed diffuse bilateral inspiratory crackles, but no wheeze. His pulse was regular at 100/min, and his blood pressure was 105/70 mmHg.

**Investigations revealed:**

haemoglobin 7.4 g/L

**Immunology:** Anti-basement membrane antibody, negative

**Sputum:** Mucoid with blood staining. Haemosiderin-laden macrophages present. No micro-organisms seen and culture negative

**Chest x-ray:** Patchy bilateral consolidation

**Lung function tests:**

| | | |
|---|---|---|
| $FEV_1$ | 1.8 L | (predicted 3) |
| FVC | 2.1 L | (predicted 3.6) |
| TLCO | 6.4 mmol/min/kPa | (NR 4.1–5.5) |
| KCO | 2.4 mmol/min/kPa | (NR 1.2–1.6) |

What is the most likely diagnosis?

A bronchiectasis

B cryptogenic fibrosing alveolitis

C extrinsic allergic alveolitis

D idiopathic pulmonary haemosiderosis

E Goodpasture's syndrome

## Question 25

A 32-year-old literary editor attends respiratory clinic with a 6 week history of chronic cough. She is a lifelong non-smoker. She denies a history of wheeze or dyspnoea, and reports no post-nasal drip syndrome. Physical examination was entirely normal. At initial attendance in clinic, she was on no medication apart from the oral contraceptive pill. Treatment of this cough with 1 week of inhaled β-agonists produced improvement, but not complete resolution, of the cough. Presence of airway hypersensitivity with the methacholine inhalation challenge was demonstrated. There was no history of antecedent illness.

The most likely diagnosis is:

A post-viral cough

B sarcoidosis

C cough-variant asthma

D ACE inhibitor therapy

E post-nasal drip syndrome

## Question 26

A 19-year-old man with a ten year history of asthma presents with a six week history of worsening symptoms of exertional breathlessness and wheeze. He has a history of eczema and hayfever as a child. He smokes 10 cigarettes a day and works as an electrician. In addition he has a cough which wakes him up most nights. The cough is unproductive. Systems review was negative, apart from some occasional diarrhoea. His current treatment is inhaled beclomethasone 800 µg per day and inhaled salbutamol 200 mcg when required via a metered dose inhaler.

Which one of the following is the next most appropriate step in management?

A add aminophylline

B add montelukast

C add salmeterol

D change to a dry powder inhaler

E double the dose of beclomethasone

## Question 27

You are asked advice by a young professional couple, Mr and Mrs X. Mrs X is nine weeks pregnant. Mr X's brother and his partner had a child with cystic fibrosis. As a result, Mr X was screened and found to carry the Δf508 mutation for cystic fibrosis. Mrs X declines to be tested.

What are the chances of Mr and Mrs X's child having cystic fibrosis, given that the gene frequency for this mutation in the general population is 1/20?

A 1/4

B 1/20

C 1/40

D 1/80

E 1/160

## Question 28

A 32-year-old man is referred to the General Medical Outpatient clinic. He and his wife had been referred by his GP to the infertility clinic for consideration for assisted conception. He is generally fit and well and works as a central heating engineer. He has been referred because he has a chronic productive cough and a history of recurrent chest infections since childhood in addition to recurrent sinusitis.

**Investigations reveal:**

| | |
|---|---|
| sodium sweat test | normal |
| serum IgG | 7.4 g/L |
| serum IgA | 1.2 g/L |
| serum IgM | 3.1 g/L |

The most likely diagnosis is:

A bronchiectasis

B Chediak-Higashi syndrome

C cystic fibrosis

D primary ciliary dyskinesia

E situs inversus

# Answers to Chapter 8: Respiratory medicine

These solutions aim to provide the reason(s) for the right answer, and also the reason(s) for the wrong answers being excluded.

1 **Answer B:** This is a factual 'best of five' question, more suited to Part 1, but the adverse prognostic factors in sarcoidosis have been known to appear in both Parts of the examination. (*See* **Learning point**.)

2 **Answer E:** This is also known as Lofgren's syndrome. It had been considered that the presentation of erythema nodosum – arthropathy – bilateral hilar lymphadenopathy is so characteristic that histological diagnosis is not necessary, but the general consensus now is that a tissue diagnosis must be attempted whenever possible, as the differential diagnosis includes TB and lymphoma. It is no longer acceptable to leave these people without further investigation. CT with HR cuts can demonstrate parenchymal changes and can direct TBBx (which results in diagnosis in up to 80% of cases). In addition, transbronchial needle aspiration of thoracic lymphadenopathy is growing in popularity (yields up to 80%), avoiding mediastinoscopy. Biopsying EN is not especially helpful as one can easily miss granuloma.

3 **Answer B:** Adequate data for LTOT prolonging survival exists only for chronic bronchitis, although in practice it is assumed to apply in other chronic hypoxaemic conditions.

4 **Answer A:** The most common symptoms are: recent onset of shortness of breath (30%), chest pain (43%), cough (35%), weight loss (23%) and increased sputum production (18%).

5 **Answer B:** Tree pollens predominate in the spring, and grass pollens (including timothy, rye, cocksfoot, meadow, dogstail) dominate in the latter part of the summer. Nettle and dock are weed pollens that peak around July and August, and fungal pollens (including *Cladosporium* and *Alternaria*) dominate in the summer too.

6 **Answer B:** ARDS is characterised by hypoxaemia, reduced lung compliance, and pulmonary infiltrates on the chest x-ray. There is damage to the capillary and endothelial cell linings, resulting in oedema and leakage of proteins into the interstitial and alveolar spaces at normal pulmonary capillary hydrostatic pressures. Wedge pressure, unlike the high pressures seen with LVF and pulmonary oedema is often normal.

7 **Answer D:** Bupropion (Zyban) is far more effective than nicotine patches in smoking cessation. However, it is contraindicated in patients with eating disorders and those with a history of seizures. There is insufficient evidence combining bupropion with nicotine patches.

8 **Answer B:** Cardiac troponins are reliable markers of myocardial injury that are being used increasingly in patients presenting with undifferentiated chest pain or dyspnoea, to diagnose an acute coronary syndrome. They also occur in patients with massive PEs because of right ventricular dilatation and myocardial injury. For acute pulmonary embolism, thrombolysis administered through a peripheral vein is as effective as through a pulmonary artery catheter. Haemoptysis is associated with pulmonary haemorrhage due to a distal clot, not a large central clot.

9 **Answer C:** Involvement of mediastinal lymph nodes is a contraindication to surgery with curative intent. It has a worse prognosis. Mediastinal nodes of greater than 1 cubic cm considered involved until proven otherwise. There is some trial data that neo-adjuvant chemotherapy can downstage some of these to allow successful surgical cure. There is also some emerging evidence for chemotherapy following 'completely' resected NSCLC. Contraindications to surgery include metastases, mediastinal LN, organ involvement, and malignant effusions. In addition, there are practical considerations in surviving thoracic surgery, most noticeably lung function. It is recommended that post BD $FEV_1$ should be > 1.5L for lobectomy and > 2L for pneumonectomy. Selected patients with worse PFT who have good oxygen saturations at rest and have undergone further assessment (TLCO, exercise testing, V/Q scanning) and have reasonable estimated postop $FEV_1$ and TLCO can be considered for surgery.

10 **Answer C:** The presence of raised serum urea (> 7 mM), hypotension (diastolic blood pressure equal or < 60 mmHg) and respiratory rate equal or > 30/min is associated with significantly increased risk of death. These are the CURB65 criteria (latest BTS guidelines).

11 **Answer B:** This lady's clinical history suggests aspiration. Her chest x-ray suggests collapse + consolidation of the right lower lobe. The lower lobes are the usual site of aspiration when the patient is upright. She may therefore have aspirated a foreign body during the choking episode and a bronchoscopy will identify this and allow removal of it.

12 **Answer A:** This lady is likely to have developed adult respiratory distress syndrome (ARDS) as a complication of her severe burns. The patient becomes tachypnoeic, increasingly breathless and cyanosed and develops refractory hypoxia. The CXR classically shows bilateral peripheral interstitial and alveolar infiltrates that become progressively more confluent but spare the costophrenic angles. Normal heart size, absent septal lines, air bronchograms and a peripheral distribution are helpful in differentiating ARDS from other conditions such as LVF.

13 **Answer D:** A HRCT scan of chest may reveal pulmonary abnormalities in sarcoidosis, such as multiple ill defined opacities running along the bronchovascular bundles, lymphatics and interlobar septa even in the absence of plain CXR abnormalities. Serum ACE is elevated in about 70% of patients with active sarcoidosis but is not sensitive or specific (it is elevated in TB, lymphoma, asbestosis and silicosis) and is therefore not helpful in diagnosis; it can however be useful to monitor progress. Histological confirmation is required to make the diagnosis with confidence. Transbronchial lung biopsy will provide positive histology in about 80% of patients, is safe and can be done under sedation with local anaesthesia, and is therefore the diagnostic investigation of choice. It is useful in demonstrating infiltration of the alveolar wells and interstitial spaces, with inflammatory cells. The Kveim test is no longer performed because of the potential risk of transmitting HIV or prion disease. Incidentally, the combination of acute sarcoidosis with erythema nodosum, oligoarthropathy and hilar lymphadenopathy normally has a good prognosis, and usually resolves spontaneously over 6–8 weeks.

14 **Answer C:** The differential diagnosis of hilar lymphadenopathy and hypercalcaemia include bronchial carcinoma, sarcoidosis, and lymphoma. The most likely diagnosis is squamous cell bronchial carcinoma, with PTHRH rather than bony metastases. Hilar involvement is usually a result of metastatic spread to the hilar nodes. CT chest is the next investigation of choice as it will help identify any further nodal involvement and allow planning of an approach to histological confirmation of the tumour.

15 **Answer B:** This clinical sign would support a diagnosis of *Mycoplasma pneumoniae.*

16 **Answer D:** This patient is otherwise well, and has no specific features of congenital heart disease such as clubbing. He appears desaturated, with saturations of 85% yet good arterial oxygen. This is a typical description of methaemoglobinaemia, which is the accumulation of reversibly oxidised methaemoglobin, causing reduced oxygen affinity of haemoglobin molecules with consequent cyanosis. The oxygen dissociation curve therefore shifts to the left. Levels below 20% produce symptoms of breathlessness and headaches, and levels above this may cause death. It can occur due to an inherited condition, or as a consequence of drugs such as nitrites. In the context of this question, however, the methaemoglobinaemia is best explained by dapsone. Other causes include chloroquine, primaquine, quinines, and sulphonamides. Methylene blue is useful in treatment.

17 **Answer B:** The patient presents with symptoms and signs that are consistent with pulmonary fibrosis. This is supported by his CXR, which shows bilateral lower zone shadowing – a reticulo-nodular pattern is seen – and his spirometry, which demonstrates a restrictive defect. His blood gases show Type 1

respiratory failure, which again is consistent with the diagnosis. HRCT of the chest is the investigation of choice. It will confirm the diagnosis of interstitial fibrosis and can be diagnostic in a number of diseases such as Usual Interstitial Pneumonia (UIP), CFA, asbestosis and sarcoidosis, preventing the need for lung biopsy. In high resolution CT, a ground-glass appearance is associated with predominantly cellular appearance on biopsy and a more active disease, which responds to treatment and has a better prognosis.

18 **Answer C:** This patient's arterial blood gases are deteriorating and he is developing an increasingly severe respiratory acidosis. He is still alert and is haemodynamically stable and therefore NIV (such as BiPAP) is the treatment of choice and should be instigated without delay (option C). Intravenous hydrocortisone (option D) would be unlikely to affect the patient's oxygen acutely, because of its duration of action. Reducing his oxygen drive (option A) would worsen his breathing. Intubation (option B) is inappropriate. Oxygen by face mask (option E), when he is already receiving 2/Litres via nasal speculae at the end of the question, would not improve his breathing.

19 **Answer D:** This patient has chronic obstructive pulmonary disease (COPD) as a result of her smoking. Her investigations demonstrate that it is severe ($FEV_1 < 40\%$ predicted). The reason why she is a candidate for long-term oxygen therapy (LTOT) is that she is hypoxic. The criteria for LTOT are $paO_2 < 7.3$ kPa (55 mmHg) with or without hypercapnia or $paO_2 < 8.0$ kPa (60 mmHg) if there is evidence of pulmonary hypertension/cor pulmonale/polycythaemia. LTOT and smoking cessation are currently the only interventions in COPD that have been shown to prolong life.

20 **Answer B:** The history and examination findings are suggestive of an interstitial lung disease (ILD), the most likely diagnosis being usual interstitial pneumonitis. The pulmonary function tests demonstrate a reduction in both $FEV_1$ and FVC ($FEV_1$/FVC = 90%) with a low diffusion capacity, i.e. restrictive defect which is consistent with ILD. The most likely diagnosis is CFA (or usual interstitial pneumonia). Bronchiectasis usually results in a productive cough and an obstructive pattern on lung function. The history and CXR findings are not suggestive of LVF and lymphangitis carcinomatosis typically produces hilar enlargement with diffuse streaky midzone infiltrates. The diagnosis can be confirmed on HRCT in most cases, although lung biopsy may be required.

21 **Answer B:** This man's lung function demonstrates an obstructive pattern. The $FEV_1$/VC is usually greater than 75% in normal young people but falls to 70–75% in normal elderly subjects. Below this is an obstructive pattern. As airway obstruction progresses both the $FEV_1$ and VC decrease. There is an increased TLC. The results also show that there is no significant reversibility to bronchodilators (i.e < 15% improvement in $FEV_1$) and the transfer co-

efficient is reduced, which is consistent with a diagnosis of COPD rather than asthma. COPD is divided into mild (FEV= 60–80%), Moderate (40–59%), and severe (< 40% predicted) (see BTS guidelines: www.brit-thoracic.org.uk).

**22 Answer B:** This lady has a history consistent with chronic obstructive airways disease. The diagnosis is confirmed on lung function; she has airways obstruction with a reduced $FEV_1$ and $FEV_1/FVC$. She has a normal total lung capacity but her residual volume is increased, indicating a degree of air trapping. Finally, her diffusion capacity (transfer factor) is decreased, which helps differentiate COPD from asthma.

**23 Answer E:** This involves tissue proliferation and infiltration by Langerhans' cells. This can be diffuse, typically in infants < 2 years, and is accompanied by a poor prognosis. It may be multifocal (as in eosinophilic granuloma, found in bone, skin, lung, meninges, and the pituitary), or localised, in which case it presents in young adult smokers and represents an unusual response to tobacco smoke.

**24 Answer D:** Idiopathic pulmonary haemosiderosis is a condition charcterised by recurrent episodes of diffuse intra-alveolar haemorrhage, associated with dyspnoea, anaemia, and sometimes fever. It is a diagnosis of exclusion, and truly idiopathic haemosiderosis is usually diagnosed in childhood. Pathology demonstrates haemosiderin-laden macrophages in the alveolar spaces and interstitium, with fibrosis developing in patients with repeated episodes of haemorrhage, and with no evidence of vasculitis. This condition can be distinguished from Goodpasture's syndrome by the absence of renal abnormalities and has a better prognosis.

**25 Answer C:** This is a history of cough-variant asthma, in effect features of asthma where the only symptom is cough. Hypersensitivity of airways with methacholine is insufficient to produce the diagnosis. It normally does not show PEFR variability. Treatment with inhaled β-agonists usually improves the symptom, although there can be a variable response; complete resolution of the cough may require up to eight weeks of therapy. Studies have demonstrated that in non-smokers who are not receiving ACE inhibitor therapy, chronic cough is accounted for by post-nasal drip syndrome, cough-variant asthma, or gastro-oesophageal reflux. Usually a 2 month trial of inhaled steroids or a short course of oral steroids will confirm a diagnosis of steroid-sensitive chronic cough (cough-variant asthma and the rare eosinophilic bronchitis).

**26 Answer C:** This patient has poorly controlled asthma. His current regime places him at step 2 of BTS guidelines but there is a clear need for an increase in therapy to control symptoms. Many RCT and meta-analyses of RCT have shown that the addition of a long acting β-agonist (LABA) such as salmeterol or eformeterol improves symptom control and lung function, and reduces exacerbations, over increasing the dose of inhaled corticosteroids, whilst other studies show clear benefits of LABA over leucotriene receptor antagonists such as montelukasts and theophyllines. See BTS/SIGN asthma guidelines in *Thorax.* 2003; **58**(Suppl. 1): 1–94.

27 **Answer D:** The chance of Mrs X being a carrier of the gene is 1/20. The chances of two carriers of a recessive gene having a child that is homozygous for that disease (i.e. both genes are transmitted to the child) is 1/4. Therefore, the chances of this couple having a child with CF are 1/4 × 1/20 = 1/80. Mutations in the CFTR gene are responsible on chromosome 7, q31.2.

28 **Answer D:** Primary ciliary dyskinesia constitutes a group of conditions that are inherited in an autosomal recessive fashion characterised by abnormal ciliary motion and impaired mucociliary clearance. The lack of effective ciliary motility causes abnormal mucociliary clearance. This leads to recurrent or persistent respiratory infections (which may lead to bronchiectasis), sinusitis, otitis media, and male infertility. In 50% of the patients, PCD is associated with situs inversus (Kartagener's syndrome), due to problems with embryonic nodal cilia leading to random assignment of laterality. The normal sweat test makes CF unlikely.

The principal differential diagnoses to consider in this case are cystic fibrosis and primary ciliary dyskinesia. The diagnosis of CF is based on typical pulmonary and/or gastrointestinal tract manifestations and positive results on sweat test (pilocarpine iontophoresis). A negative sweat test is sufficient evidence to exclude CF as a diagnostic possibility. While the patient may have bronchiectasis, this alone is not sufficient to account for his other symptoms. In the exam, as well, watch out for hypogammaglobulinaemia masquerading as CF.

# Learning Points

## *Question 1*

### Learning point

**Adverse prognostic factors in sarcoidosis include:**

Age of onset > 40 years
Black race
Cardiac involvement
Chronic hypercalcaemia
Chronic uveitis
Cystic bone lesions
Lupus pernio
Nasal mucosal involvement
Nephrocalcinosis
Neurosarcoidosis
Progressive pulmonary fibrosis

## CHAPTER 9

# Nephrology

Renal medicine for the MRCP is usually given a lot of weight. This is because there is a lot to examine, including basic glomerular and tubular disorders, infections of the kidney (and particularly reflux nephropathy), stone formation, acute and chronic renal failure, hypertension and renal problems in pregnancy, the effects of drugs on the kidney, and the different types of dialysis modalities and their complications (including problems with immunosuppression) – in relation to 'renal replacement therapy'.

### NORMAL VALUES (BLOOD)

| | | |
|---|---|---|
| complement component | $C_3$ | 60–180 mg/dL |
| complement component | $C_4$ | 10–35 mg/dL |
| immunoglobulins | IgG | 6–13 g/L |
| | IgA | 0.8–3.7 g/L |
| | IgM | 0.4–2.2 g/L |

# Questions

## Question 1

A 69-year-old male is diagnosed with nephrotic syndrome. He receives steroid therapy without benefit.

| **Investigations reveal:** | |
|---|---|
| serum albumin | 20 g/L |
| serum total cholesterol | 12 mmol/L |
| **Urinalysis:** | protein (+++) |
| **Renal biopsy:** | focal segmental glomerulosclerosis |

Which one of the following steps is most likely to preserve renal function?

A dietary salt restriction

B low dietary protein intake

C ramipril

D simvastatin

E warfarin

## Question 2

A 79-year-old lady presents to her GP. Her previous medical history includes a chronic discharging sinus relating to a hip operation 10 years previously. Her medications include naproxen and flucloxacillin, as well as paracetamol (as required) for intermittent forearm pains. Examination reveals pitting oedema to mid-shins and a 3 cm liver edge.

Investigations: serum sodium 138 mmol/L, serum potassium 4.4 mmol/L, serum creatinine 520 µmol/L, serum albumin 32 g/L, serum alkaline phosphatase 270 U/L, serum calcium 2.3 mmol/L, haemoglobin 10.8 g/L, white cell count 9.2 × 109/L, immunoglobulins: IgA 3.8 g/L, IgG 19 g/L, IgM 2.0 g/L. 24-hour urinary protein collection was 3.8g. KUB ultrasound revealed normal sized kidneys.

The most likely diagnosis is:

A multiple myeloma

B analgesic nephropathy

C AL amyloidosis

D AA amyloidosis

E acute tubulo-interstitial nephritis

## Question 3

A 68-year-old woman presented to her GP. She was found to have symptoms and signs of active synovitis, with elevated inflammatory markers. She had been taking IM sodium aurothiomalate 50 mg once a week for the previous six months. Other medications included diclofenac 50 mg three times a day. She had well controlled ischaemic heart disease and recent onset atrial fibrillation. Her medications also included aspirin 75 mg, recently changed to warfarin. Her renal function, measured a month previously, had been normal.

**Recent investigations revealed:**

| **Blood tests:** | |
|---|---|
| serum sodium | 138 mmol/L |
| serum potassium | 4.9 mmol/L |
| serum urea | 12.9 mmol/L |
| serum creatinine | 290 µmol/L |

| **Further tests:** | |
|---|---|
| **Urinalysis:** | protein (++), blood (++) |
| **24-hour urine collection:** | 0.4 g protein/day |

What is the most likely cause for her deterioration in renal function?

A amyloidosis

B gold nephropathy

C interstitial nephritis

D multiple myeloma

E vasculitis

## Question 4

A 58-year-old man attends a Well Man Clinic because his father died of a heart attack in his early 60s. There is no past history of diabetes mellitus, but he is a smoker of 15–20 cigarettes per day. On examination, he has a BMI of 28 kg/m$^2$ and has a blood pressure of 162/88 mmHg. Cardiovascular, chest and abdominal examination are normal. Fundoscopy shows AV nipping. He is advised to reattend his GP, who confirms the sustained elevation in blood pressure with recordings averaging 170/94 mmHg.

**Investigations reveal:**

**Blood tests:**

| | |
|---|---|
| serum sodium | 144 mmol/L |
| serum potassium | 4.2 mmol/L |
| serum urea | 12.6 mmol/L |
| serum creatinine | 186 µmol/L |
| random plasma glucose | 10.1 mmol/L |
| HbA1c | 7% |
| serum total cholesterol | 6.8 mmol/L |
| serum triglycerides | 2.6 mmol/L |
| **Urinary dipstix:** | protein (+) |
| **Ultrasound of the kidneys:** | normal size |

What is the most likely cause of his renal impairment?

A analgesic nephropathy

B chronic glomerulonephritis

C diabetic nephropathy

D hypertensive nephropathy

E renovascular disease

## Question 5

A 60-year-old man presented with a three day history of malaise, fevers and feet ulceration. He had given up jogging recently due to newly-diagnosed angina. He was then found to have a stenotic aortic valve and diffuse moderate triple vessel disease. He underwent an aortic valve replacement, which helped initially, but his symptoms deteriorated recently. His sister has type II diabetes mellitus. His medication was atenolol, slow release nifedipine, isosorbide mononitrate and warfarin. He previously smoked around 35 cigarettes/day, but gave up after his surgery. He enjoyed three pints of beer every evening. On examination, several toes demonstrated ulceration, dusky blue in appearance, and he had livedo reticularis. He was afebrile, his pulse was 60/min, blood pressure 190/110, there was a mechanical second heart sound with an opening click and a soft ejection systolic murmur. Good peripheral pulses were palpable. There was no organomegaly.

**Investigations revealed:**

| | |
|---|---|
| **Blood tests:** | |
| haemoglobin | 10.5 g/L |
| white blood cells | $13.9 \times 10^9$/L (3% eosinophils) |
| serum sodium | 139 mmol/L |
| serum potassium | 4.4 mmol/L |
| serum urea | 26.8 mmol/L |
| serum creatinine | 311 µmol/L |
| serum alanine amino transferase | 123 U/L |
| serum albumin | 36 g/L |
| serum globulin | 78 g/L |
| **Immunology:** | ANA, ANCA, anti-dsDNA, anti-cardiolipin antibodies negative. |
| **Blood cultures:** | three sets – all negative |
| **Urinary dipstix:** | protein (++), red cells (+) |
| **Urine microscopy:** | red cells, occasional hyaline cast |
| **Chest x-ray:** | normal lung fields, normal heart |
| **TTE:** | well-seated prosthetic aortic valve. No vegetations seen. |

The most likely diagnosis is:

A vasculitis

B polyarteritis nodosa

C cholesterol emboli

D Churg-Strauss syndrome

E infective endocarditis

## Question 6

A 28-year-old woman who attended for contraceptive advice three months post partum was found to be hypertensive. She had a recent history of lethargy, aphthous ulceration and painful extremities in the cold. She had no past medical history of note and took no medications. On examination, she had a temperature of 37.4°C, her wrists were noted to be warm and swollen, she had mild diffuse alopecia, blood pressure was 180/108 with Grade II retinopathy, the apex beat was not displaced, she had a grade 2/6 ejection-systolic murmur and all other systems were normal.

Investigations revealed: serum sodium 139 units, serum potassium 5.4 units, serum creatinine 212 units, serum total bilirubin 25 units, LDH 910 (270–620 iU/L), serum albumin 32 g/L, haemoglobin 8.4 g/L, white cell count $3.1 \times 10^9$/L, platelet count $95 \times 10^9$/L, PTT 14 s. Urinalysis revealed: protein (++), blood (++), white and red cell casts. KUB and ultrasound of the kidneys and renal tract were normal, and echocardiogram was normal. Blood cultures revealed coagulase negative *Staphylococcus* in one bottle (of two).

The most likely diagnosis is:

**A** infective endocarditis

**B** microscopic polyangiitis

**C** systemic lupus erythematosus

**D** post-streptococcal glomerulonephritis

**E** HELLP syndrome

## Question 7

A 40-year-old male underwent an elective ERCP for a common bile duct stone. Post ERCP, he developed acute septicaemia. Biochemistry pre- and post-ERCP is shown below. He is diaphoretic, flushed and tachycardic (125 beats per minute). The blood pressure is 85/55 mmHg and he is producing 10 mL of urine per hour.

| | *Pre-ERCP* | *Post-ERCP* |
|---|---|---|
| serum sodium (mmol/L) | 136 | 140 |
| serum potassium (mmol/L) | 4 | 4 |
| serum chloride (mmol/L) | 100 | 103 |
| serum bicarbonate (mmol/L) | 28 | 20 |
| serum urea (mmol/L) | 4 | 40 |
| serum creatinine (µmol/L) | 96 | 720 |

Based on recent clinical trials, which one of the following management steps has been shown to improve survival?

A give high dose frusemide (furosemide)

B give low dose dopamine

C give low dose dopamine, frusemide (furosemide) and mannitol

D give frusemide (furosemide) and mannitol

E none of the above

## Question 8

A 65-year-old man develops oliguria 24 hours after a Dacron repair of an abdominal aortic aneurysm. The blood pressure is 115/95 and a chest x-ray shows no evidence of infection or oedema.

**Serum electrolytes reveal:**

| | |
|---|---|
| sodium | 145 mmol/L |
| potassium | 4.6 mmol/L |
| urea | 14.5 mmol/L |
| creatinine | 129 µmol/L |
| plasma osmolality | 289 mOsm/kg |

The most sensible initial step is:

A administration of a fluid challenge

B measurement of urine sodium

C measurement of the ratio of urine to plasma osmolality

D calculation of the fractional sodium excretion

E insertion of a Swann-Ganz catheter

## Question 9

A 22-year-old man was admitted with a two-day history of nausea and blood-stained diarrhoea. He recalled having eaten a beef and horseradish sandwich from a local corner shop three days previously. On examination, he was febrile (38.4°C) and there was periorbital oedema. The blood pressure was 150/90 mmHg. His abdomen was soft, but tender.

| **Investigations revealed:** | |
|---|---|
| haemoglobin | 8.4 g/L |
| white cell count | $13 \times 10^9$/L |
| platelet count | $36 \times 10^9$/L |
| prothrombin time | 13 s |
| APTT | 34 s |
| serum sodium | 138 mmol/L |
| serum potassium | 5.9 mmol/L |
| serum urea | 13 mmol/L |
| serum creatinine | 150 µmol/L |
| **Blood film:** | red cell fragments |

What is the most appropriate investigation to secure the diagnosis?

A blood cultures

B stool sample for *E. coli* 0157:H7

C stool sample for parasites, ova and cysts

D urine culture

E urine microscopy

## Question 10

A patient with chronic renal failure, treated with regular haemodialysis, attends the renal clinic. He has been treated for six months with oral ferrous sulphate, 200 mg three times a day but admits to poor compliance with this treatment. His haemoglobin at this clinic attendance is 7.6, with an MCV of 88 fL and a serum ferritin of 32 µg/L.

Which of the following is the most appropriate treatment?

A blood transfusion

B commence subcutaneous erythropoietin

C increase the dose of oral ferrous sulphate

D intravenous iron

E intravenous iron and subcutaneous erythropoietin

## Question 11

A 45-year-old lady with chronic renal failure secondary to systemic lupus erythematosus is seen in a renal clinic as a routine follow up. Her joints have been causing some discomfort and she has been taking naproxen as required, as well as prednisolone 2.5 mg od with azathioprine 50 mg od for disease control. She has stable renal function with a serum creatinine of 300 μmol/L and a serum creatinine clearance of 18 mL/min. Associated with her chronic renal failure she has controlled secondary hyperparathyroidism. She has been anaemic for the last six months and investigation of dyspepsia with an endoscopy showed only mild gastritis. She has already been on oral ferrous sulphate 200 mg tds for three months.

**Investigations reveal:**

| | |
|---|---|
| haemoglobin | 9.4 g/L |
| [hypochromic red cells | 12%] |
| platelet count | 180 × $10^9$/L |
| white cell count | 6.4 × $10^9$/L |
| serum folate | 4.0 μg/L |
| serum ferritin | 230 ng/L |
| transferrin saturation | 17% |

What therapeutic intervention should now be considered?

A folate

B GM-CSF

C intravenous iron

D subcutaneous erythropoietin

E vitamin $B_{12}$

## Question 12

A 78-year-old diabetic man, on regular haemodialysis (four hours three times a week) for 12 years presents with increasing bilateral shoulder pain, hand pain associated with stiffness and numbness. His lower limbs are not affected. His medications include calcium carbonate two tablets three times a day with meals, ACE inhibitor, aspirin and 1-alpha-calcidol 1 μg once a day. Which of the following explanations may best account for his symptoms?

A aluminium toxicity

B amyloidosis

C cerebrovascular disease due to antithrombin III deficiency

D diabetic neuropathy

E uraemia

## Question 13

A 68-year-old man has dialysis via a tunnelled haemodialysis catheter. He is seen on the renal unit complaining of general malaise. He is complaining of shortness of breath and tiredness, has lost weight over the last four months and is not sleeping well, due to sweats. Sometimes he has joint aches and back pain which are mainly lumbar in origin. The back pain is getting worse but does not stop him mobilising. He had a course of flucloxacillin for an infection of his dialysis line four weeks previously, and this appeared to clear the infection. He has dialysis three times per week for four hours per session and has had no recorded pyrexias. He takes a combination of calcium carbonate tablets and Alucaps for hyperphosphataemia, which is now controlled. His aluminium levels are normal and his plasma parathyroid hormone level is only mildly elevated, 1-alpha-calcidol having been started. He has been on erythropoietin for six months and receives intravenous iron on dialysis days.

On examination, he is apyrexial and has normal heart sounds, with a clear chest and no pulmonary oedema. Abdomen is soft and non-tender. Rectal examination is normal. He has some lumbar spine tenderness.

**Investigations reveal:**

| | |
|---|---|
| haemoglobin | 7.8 g/L |
| MCV | 85 fl |
| white cell count | $8.0 \times 10^9$/L |
| platelet count | $180 \times 10^9$/L |
| erythrocyte sedimentation rate | 78 mm in the 1st hour |
| serum ferritin | 777 µg/L |
| serum C-reactive protein | 125 mg/L |

What is the most likely cause of his unresponsiveness to erythropoietin?

A aluminium toxicity

B sepsis

C hypersplenism

D hyperparathyroidism

E occult gastrointestinal bleeding

## Question 14

A 32-year-old woman is seen in the Outpatient clinic three weeks after receiving a cadaveric renal transplant. She is currently taking prednisolone and ciclosporin. Three days ago her serum urea and electrolytes were normal. She says that she feels well and a trough ciclosporin level is satisfactory. Repeat serum urea and electrolytes show:

| | |
|---|---|
| serum sodium | 139 mmol/L |
| serum potassium | 3.9 mmol/L |
| serum urea | 11 mmol/L |
| serum creatinine | 168 µmol/L |

The renal transplant was HLA matched.

The patient was CMV IgG negative; the kidney donor was CMV IgG positive.

Which of the following best accounts for the change in renal function?

A acute cellular rejection

B ciclosporin toxicity

C CMV infection

D dehydration

E pyelonephritis of the transplanted kidney

## Question 15

A 62-year-old male smoker presented to the emergency department with acute dyspnoea. His previous medical history included three vessel coronary artery bypass surgery for ischaemic heart disease and hypertension. Examination revealed hypertension and widespread expiratory crackles. A chest x-ray confirmed the presence of pulmonary oedema. He was treated with intravenous nitrates and frusemide (furosemide) with symptomatic improvement. He was put on oral frusemide (furosemide) at a dose of 80 mg (od) and captopril 12.5 mg bd and his bloods were checked one week later.

| | *Initially (on presentation)* | *After a week of treatment* |
|---|---|---|
| serum sodium (mmol/L) | 138 | 134 |
| serum potassium (mmol/L) | 4.2 | 5.4 |
| serum urea (mmol/L) | 8.7 | 15.7 |
| serum creatinine (μmol/L) | 170 | 220 |
| fasting plasma glucose (mmol/L) | 6.0 | |
| **Urinalysis:** | protein (++) | |

What is the most likely cause of his deterioration in renal function?

A captopril

B cholesterol emboli

C diabetic nephropathy

D frusemide (furosemide)

E hypertension

## Question 16

A 78-year-old hypertensive woman is admitted to hospital with an acute coronary syndrome. Six days later, having made a good recovery, she is discharged on atenolol 50 mg, enalapril 10 mg, isosorbide mononitrate 30 mg, atorvastatin 20 mg and aspirin 75 mg daily. Her investigations at admission revealed a serum urea concentration of 12.4 mmol/L with a serum creatinine of 250 μmol/L. Her electrolytes are checked one week later with the following results:

| | |
|---|---|
| serum sodium | 143 mmol/L |
| serum potassium | 6.1 mmol/L |
| serum bicarbonate | 18 mmol/L |
| serum urea | 28.9 mmol/L |
| serum creatinine | 410 μmol/L |

She is well, but agrees to return to hospital. An ECG shows T wave inversion in leads II, III, V5 and V6. A chest x-ray shows moderate cardiomegaly but is otherwise normal.

What is the best course of action?

A calcium resonium

B haemodialysis

C insulin and dextrose infusion

D sodium bicarbonate infusion

E stop enalapril and recheck U & Es in 12 hours

## Question 17

A 50-year-old male presents with a 4 week history of exertional shortness of breath. Two years previously he had been diagnosed by his GP with asthma, for which he was prescribed a salbutamol inhaler, and he has been taking ibuprofen over the last six months for arthritis of the hips. Two weeks previously he returned from a 6 week holiday in Thailand. Examination reveals a rather ill-looking and tanned individual with a temperature of 37°C, a blood pressure of 146/86 mmHg and a heart rate of 106/min. There are scattered bibasal fine crackles with occasional wheeze on chest examination, and a left-sided foot drop.

| **Investigations reveal:** | |
|---|---|
| haemoglobin | 14 g/L |
| white cell count | $8.8 \times 10^9$/L |
| neutrophil count | $3.5 \times 10^9$/L |
| lymphocyte count | $2 \times 10^9$/L |
| monocyte count | $0.1 \times 10^9$/L |
| eosinophil count | $1.6 \times 10^9$/L |
| platelet count | $528 \times 10^9$/L |
| erythrocyte sedimentation rate | 65 mm/hr (Westergren) |
| serum sodium | 136 mmol/L |
| serum potassium | 7.0 mmol/L |
| serum chloride | 106 mmol/L |
| serum bicarbonate | 15 mmol/L |
| serum creatinine | 320 µmol/L |

| **Further tests:** | |
|---|---|
| **Immunology:** | anti-proteinase 3 positive |
| **Ultrasound of the kidneys:** | right kidney 12 cm, left kidney 13 cm<br>no obstruction seen |
| **Urinalysis:** | protein (++), blood (+++) |

What is the most likely diagnosis?

A amyloidosis

B analgesic nephropathy

C Churg-Strauss syndrome

D membranous glomerulonephritis

E mesangiocapillary glomerulonephritis type II

## Question 18

A 22-year-old female was admitted to hospital three days after the onset of a sore throat. The patient also complained of abdominal pain, loose stools, and wrist and ankle pain. On examination, there was a non-blanching rash over the back, buttocks and lower legs (particularly shins and thighs). Her blood pressure was 175/90 mmHg.

**Investigations revealed:**

| | |
|---|---|
| serum urea | 8 mmol/L |
| serum creatinine | 118 μmol/L |
| serum albumin | 30 g/L |
| **Urinalysis:** | protein (++), blood (+) |

What is the best initial treatment?

A ACE inhibitor

B azathioprine

C cyclophosphamide

D high dose prednisolone

E plasma exchange

## Questions 19 and 20

These results below were obtained on a 52-year-old lady with a history of recurrent urinary tract infections. Ten years previously, she had a total colectomy for pancolitis. Her only medication was immodium.

| **Investigations revealed:** | |
|---|---|
| serum sodium | 147 mmol/L |
| serum potassium | 3.4 mmol/L |
| serum bicarbonate | 17 mmol/L |
| serum urea | 16.5 mmol/L |
| serum creatinine | 288 µmol/L |
| serum calcium (corrected) | 2.4 mmol/L |
| serum phosphate | 1.6 mmol/L |
| serum alkaline phosphatase | 120 U/L |
| serum urate | 0.4 mmol/L |
| **Urinalysis:** | serial cultures: *E. coli* |
| | urate normal |
| | pH 5.3 |

## Question 19

What is the most likely cause of her recurrent UTIs?

A oxalate stones

B fistula to bowel

C urate stones

D idiopathic hypercalciuria

E ureteric reflux

## Question 20

What single investigation should be performed?

A plain KUB x-ray

B intravenous urography

C barium enema

D barium meal

E micturating cystourethrogram

## Question 21

A 27-year-old woman is seen in clinic for investigation of lower abdominal discomfort. She has been aware of vague abdominal discomfort for many months, with dysuria, which has occurred intermittently. Her weight has been generally steady although occasionally she loses her appetite. She has otherwise been well and is married, with a child. Her only medication is the combined oral contraceptive pill, which she has been taking for many years. Examination reveals a well-looking woman with a BMI of 24.5 kg/m$^2$ and a blood pressure of 140/80 mmHg. No specific abnormalities are noted on chest, heart or abdominal examination. No abnormal neurology is noted and fundoscopic examination is normal. An ultrasonic examination of the abdomen shows only a small right kidney. Her serum urea is 5.9 mmol/L with a serum creatinine concentration of 90 µmol/L. Dipstick testing of the urine reveals blood (+), protein (+).

What is the most likely cause of this patient's presentation?

**A** chronic glomerulonephritis

**B** congenital renal atrophy

**C** fibromuscular dysplasia

**D** IgA nephropathy

**E** reflux nephropathy

## Question 22

A 39-year-old man was referred to the renal clinic. Two weeks previously he had an episode of loin pain, and passed a small renal stone. Analysis of the stone had shown it to contain mostly calcium. He is initially advised to increase his fluid intake, but he then returns to your clinic after one month. He had one previous episode, three years before, but did not seek medical advice. He was otherwise fit and well.

**Investigations revealed:**

| **Blood tests:** | |
|---|---|
| haemoglobin | 14.5 g/L |
| white blood cells | $7.5 \times 10^9$/L |
| platelet count | $210 \times 10^9$/L |
| serum sodium | 137 mmol/L |
| serum potassium | 4.2 mmol/L |
| serum urea | 6.1 mmol/L |
| serum creatinine | 100 µmol/L |
| serum corrected calcium | 2.3 mmol/L |

| **Further tests:** | |
|---|---|
| 24-hour urine volume: | 1150 mL/day |
| 24-hour urinary calcium collection: | 18 mmol/day |

Which of the following medications are likely to be of benefit?

A allopurinol

B furosemide (frusemide)

C potassium bicarbonate

D potassium citrate

E bendrofluazide (bendroflumethiazide)

## Questions 23 and 24

A 55-year-old keen gardener presents with left loin pain. His pain radiates to the groin from his left loin and is severe in nature, coming in spasms. He has previously had a resection of small bowel with a jejunocolic anastomosis for Crohn's disease. Prior to admission he had been eating well with a normal diet, high in fibre, and usually he drinks 3 litres of fluid per day. His Crohn's disease had been quiescent on steroids for the last twelve months. His nutritional history includes a good intake of vegetables from his allotment, and his bowel habit is normal for him, with two loose stools per day. His regular medication includes azathioprine, 150 mg daily.

On examination, his pulse is 96 beats per minute, and his blood pressure is 180/70 mmHg. His abdomen is soft, but he is tender in the left loin.

**Investigations reveal:**

| | |
|---|---|
| **Urinalysis:** | blood (+++), no protein, no nitrites |
| **Urine microscopy:** | no white cells or organisms |
| **Urine pH:** | 5.5. |
| **Radiology:** | A plain abdominal kidney/ureter/bladder (KUB) x-ray show a radio-opaque area over the left ureter. An intravenous urogram (IVU) confirms the presence of a small calculus. |

## Question 23

What is the most likely cause of his renal stone?

A struvite

B cysteine

C calcium oxalate

D urate

E xanthine

## Question 24

Which of the following interventions would be most effective in preventing further renal calculi?

A allopurinol

B dietary exclusion of beetroot, spinach and rhubarb

C increase daily oral fluid intake

D regular lithotripsy

E thiazide diuretic

## Question 25

A 25-year-old female presents for annual review. She developed diabetes mellitus at the age of 15 and currently is treated with human mixed insulin twice daily. Over the last one year she has been aware of episodes of dysuria and has received treatment with trimethoprim on 4 separate occasions for cystitis.

Examination reveals no specific abnormality except for two dot haemorrhages bilaterally on fundal examination. Her blood pressure is 116/76 mmHg.

**Investigations reveal:**

**Blood tests:**

| | |
|---|---|
| HbA1c | 9% |
| fasting plasma glucose | 12.1 mmol/L |
| serum sodium | 138 mmol/L |
| serum potassium | 3.6 mmol/L |
| serum urea | 4.5 mmol/L |
| serum creatinine | 90 µmol/L |

**Further tests:**

| | |
|---|---|
| **Urinalysis:** | glucose (+) |
| **24-hour urinary protein collection:** | 220 mg/day |

There is good data from randomised, controlled trials to support which of the following management steps in this patient?

A improve glycaemic control with more aggressive insulin therapy

B improve glycaemic control with more aggressive insulin therapy and start an ACE inhibitor

C start an ACE inhibitor

D give a low protein diet

E treat with prolonged antibiotics

## Question 26

A 55-year-old male consulted his general practitioner with a three month history of lethargy and weight loss. Six years previously, he had been diagnosed with diabetes mellitus and was receiving glibenclamide 10 mg daily and metformin 1g twice daily. On examination he was noted to have a BMI of 25.6 kg/m$^2$, a pulse of 88/min and a blood pressure of 164/102 mmHg. Fundal examination revealed numerous dot haemorrhages in the temporal retina of both eyes, with occasional hard exudates. Loss of position and vibration sensation were also noted to the mid shins bilaterally.

| **Investigations revealed:** | |
|---|---|
| haemoglobin | 12 g/L |
| white cell count | 4.8 × 10$^9$/L |
| serum platelet count | 195 × 10$^9$/L |
| serum sodium | 137 mmol/L |
| serum potassium | 4.6 mmol/L |
| serum urea | 16.7 mmol/L |
| serum creatinine | 220 μmol/L |
| HbA1c | 9.3% |
| **Urinalysis:** | protein (++), blood (+), ketones (+) |

What is the next best management step?

**A** change glibenclamide to insulin

**B** maximise his current oral hypoglycaemic therapy

**C** start rosiglitazone

**D** stop metformin

**E** stop metformin and glibenclamide and start insulin

## Question 27

A 19-year-old woman is seen following recurrent episodes of cystitis, despite trimethoprim therapy. She was diagnosed with diabetes mellitus at the age of 12 and now receives twice daily mixed insulin. She has taken the oral contraceptive pill for the last two years and smokes 10 cigarettes daily. She has two elder brothers who are both well. Examination reveals a thin but well looking female with a BMI of 21.5 kg/m$^2$, a blood pressure of 108/76 mmHg and normal cardiovascular, respiratory and abdominal examinations.

**Investigations reveal:**

| | |
|---|---|
| serum sodium | 140 mmol/L |
| serum potassium | 4.5 mmol/L |
| serum urea | 5.6 mmol/L |
| serum creatinine | 95 μmol/L |
| fasting plasma glucose | 10.2 mmol/L |
| HbA1c | 10.1% |

Ultrasound of the kidneys suggests reflux nephropathy.

What is the best treatment to preserve her renal function?

A ACE inhibitor

B prophylactic antibiotics

C stop smoking

D strict glycaemic control

E surgical intervention to correct reflux

## Question 28

A 58-year-old male with a three month history of lethargy and weight loss was reviewed by his GP. He had a ten year history of type 2 diabetes for which he was treated with glibenclamide 10 mg daily and metformin 1 gm twice daily. He was receiving amlodipine 10 mg daily as treatment for his hypertension. He confessed to poor compliance with diet, he smoked around five cigarettes daily, and drank approximately 12 units of alcohol per week. On examination, he was noted to have a BMI of 25.6 kg/m$^2$, a pulse of 88/min (regular), and a blood pressure of 164/102 mmHg. Fundal examination revealed dot haemorrhages in the temporal retina of both eyes, with occasional hard exudates. Loss of position and vibration sensation were also noted to the mid tibia bilaterally. Peripheral pulses were all preserved.

**Investigations revealed:**

| | |
|---|---|
| haemoglobin | 11.5 g/L |
| white cell count | 4.8 × 10$^9$/L |
| platelet count | 195 × 10$^9$/L |
| serum sodium | 137 mmol/L |
| serum potassium | 4.6 mmol/L |
| serum urea | 16.7 mmol/L |
| serum creatinine | 220 μmol/L |
| HbA1c | 9.3% |
| **Urinalysis:** | protein (++), blood (+) |

What is the most appropriate treatment for this patient's blood pressure?

A ACE inhibitor and further antihypertensives if needed to keep BP < 150/90

B ACE inhibitor and further antihypertensives if needed to keep BP < 140/80

C increase antihypertensives (but exclude ACE inhibitor) to keep BP < 150/90

D increase antihypertensives (but exclude ACE inhibitor) to keep BP < 140/80

E lifestyle advice

## Question 29

A 26-year-old female who is 13 weeks pregnant is seen in the Outpatient clinic and noted to have a sustained blood pressure of 170/92 mmHg. She has no past medical history of note, and has otherwise been well and asymptomatic. This is her first pregnancy. Examination is otherwise normal and no abnormalities are noted on fundoscopy. Ultrasound examination of the kidneys shows both kidneys to be of normal size. Urinalysis reveals protein (++) and blood (+). What is the most likely cause of her hypertension?

A pre-eclampsia

B IgA nephropathy

C fibromuscular dysplasia

D membranous nephropathy

E reflux nephropathy

## Question 30

A 34-year-old man was admitted to hospital with macroscopic haematuria. He had recently arrived in London from Nigeria. He was not taking any medications, and denied any other symptoms. On examination, his blood pressure was 130/80 mmHg.

| **Investigations revealed:** | |
|---|---|
| haemoglobin | 11.5 g/L |
| MCV | 68 fL |
| reticulocyte count | 4% |
| serum sodium | 136 mmol/L |
| serum potassium | 3.9 mmol/L |
| serum urea | 7.9 mmol/L |
| serum creatinine | 130 µmol/L |
| serum C-reactive protein | 8 mg/L |
| **Urinalysis:** | protein (+), blood (+++) |

What is the most likely cause of the haematuria?

A analgesic nephropathy

B renal vein thrombosis

C renal papillary necrosis

D *Plasmodium* infection

E pyelonephritis

## Question 31

Which of the following is most strongly associated with minimal change glomerulonephropathy?

A lead exposure

B Hodgkin's disease

C penicillamine

D mercury exposure

E cadmium exposure

## Question 32

A 34-year-old man was referred to the renal clinic. He had noticed some mild facial swelling and increasing swelling of his ankles over the previous six weeks. His blood pressure was 170/100 mmHg. Initial investigations by his GP showed:

| | |
|---|---|
| serum sodium | 140 mmol/L |
| serum potassium | 5.0 mmol/L |
| serum urea | 12 mmol/L |
| serum creatinine | 128 µmol/L |
| serum albumin | 22 g/L |
| urinary dipstix | protein (++++), blood (+) |
| **24-hour urinary protein:** | 9 g/day |

Six weeks after prednisolone (60 mg od) was commenced, a 24-hour urinary collection was repeated, demonstrating a protein content of 0.7 g/day.

Which of the following would be most likely to be seen upon renal biopsy?

A antiglomerular basement membrane disease

B IgA glomerulonephritis

C membranous glomerulonephritis

D mesangiocapillary glomerulonephritis

E minimal change glomerulonephritis

## Question 33

A 43-year-old man has had vague malaise for three weeks. Physical examination is normal, except for a blood pressure of 150/95 mmHg and pitting oedema of the legs to the knees. Dipstix urinalysis shows protein (+++) but no glucose, blood, ketones, nitrite or urobilinogen. Additional laboratory testing reveals a 24-hour urine protein of 4.1 g/day. His serum creatinine is 100 µmol/L. Liver function is normal; however, his hepatitis B surface antigen test is positive.

Which of the following conditions is he most likely to have?

A membranous glomerulonephritis

B systemic lupus erythematosus

C acute tubular necrosis

D diabetic nephropathy

E post-streptococcal glomerulonephritis

## Question 34

A 19-year-old female patient presents with gross oedema and frothy urine. She is investigated and is found to have a serum albumin of 10 g/L and heavy proteinuria of 11.5 g/day with a cholesterol of 9 mmol/L. She undergoes a renal biopsy and a diagnosis of minimal change nephropathy is made. She initially goes into remission with oral prednisolone but, on withdrawal of steroids, she is readmitted with a painful left leg and further significant oedema of the arms, legs and face. A deep vein thrombosis extending to her left external iliac vein is diagnosed on Doppler ultrasonography. She is commenced on intravenous heparin (5000 U intravenous bolus followed by infusion of 15 U/kg/h increased after six hours to 18 U/kg/h) but her left leg swelling fails to respond and 36 hours later the following results are obtained:

| | |
|---|---|
| serum albumin | 14 g/L |
| APTT ratio | 1.2 |
| international normalised ratio | 1.3 |

What is the most likely cause of these results?

A inadequate heparin

B protein C deficiency

C factor V Leiden mutation

D antithrombin III deficiency

E antiphospholipid syndrome

## Question 35

A moderately obese 16-year-old girl was referred with abdominal swelling, ankle oedema and weight gain. The blood pressure was 140/90 mmHg.

**Investigations revealed:**

| | |
|---|---|
| haemoglobin | 10.5 g/L |

Which investigation should be performed next?

A 24-hour urinary protein estimation

B abdominal ultrasound

C plasma protein electrophoresis

D urinary beta-human chorionic gonadotrophin

E urinary albumin:creatinine ratio

## Question 36

A 9-year-old girl presented to you, by her mother, has a two week history of deteriorating puffiness of the face. She has been aware of tiredness and lethargy over the last two months since having acquired a throat infection. Over this period she has gained at least 5 kg in weight. She was previously well and she takes no medication. Examination reveals generalised puffiness with pitting oedema of the lower limbs. Her blood pressure is 133/86 mmHg with a pulse of 88/min. Chest, cardiovascular and abdominal examinations are normal. Her urinary dipstick produces (+++) protein, but no blood.

**Other investigations reveal:**

| | |
|---|---|
| haemoglobin | 14 g/L |
| white cell count | $6 \times 10^9$/L |
| platelet count | $250 \times 10^9$/L |
| serum sodium | 136 mmol/L |
| serum potassium | 4.0 mmol/L |
| serum chloride | 103 mmol/L |
| serum bicarbonate | 24 mmol/L |
| serum urea | 4.2 mmol/L |
| serum creatinine | 68 µmol/L |
| serum albumin | 25 g/L |
| **24-hour urinary protein:** | 4.3 g/L |

What is the best treatment for this patient?

A observe

B intravenous serum albumin

C intravenous frusemide (furosemide)

D oral prednisolone

E oral cyclophosphamide

## Question 37

A 65-year-old woman, previously fit and well on no medications, was admitted with an intracranial bleed under the care of the neurosurgeons. Following magnetic resonance angiography, she underwent clipping of a cerebral arterial aneurysm and made a good neurological recovery postoperatively. No diuretics were administered and the following blood chemistry results on successive postoperative days were documented:

| | *Day 1* | *Day 2* | *Day 3* | *Day 4* |
|---|---|---|---|---|
| serum sodium (mmol/L) | 130 | 127 | 124 | 120 |
| serum potassium (mmol/L) | 3.5 | 3.4 | 3.4 | 3.5 |
| serum urea (mmol/L) | 4.2 | 5.1 | 5.8 | 6.8 |
| serum creatinine (μmol/L) | 70 | 78 | 75 | 88 |

On day 4 the heart rate was 92 bpm and blood pressure was 115/75 mmHg lying and 102/60 mmHg sitting up.

**Further investigations revealed:**

| | |
|---|---|
| serum osmolality | 251 mOsmol/kg |
| serum uric acid | 296 μmol/L |
| urine sodium | 80 mmol/L |
| urine osmolality | 211 mOsmol/kg |
| 24-hour urine collection | 4000 mL |

What is the most likely diagnosis?

A cranial diabetes inspidus

B hypoadrenalism

C fluid overload

D syndrome of inappropriate ADH (SIADH)

E cerebral salt wasting syndrome

## Question 38

A 52-year-old man with small-cell lung carcinoma presents with two generalised tonic clonic seizures, 1 hour apart, following a one day history of increasing lethargy, confusion and drowsiness. He is clinically euvolaemic and there are no focal neurological signs, although he is drowsy and poorly cooperative.

**Investigations reveal:**

| | |
|---|---|
| serum sodium | 108 mmol/L |
| serum potassium | 3.9 mmol/L |
| serum urea | 7.5 mmol/L |
| serum creatinine | 44 µmol/L |
| BM stix | 5.2 mmol/L |
| urine osmolality | 600 mOsmol/kg |

Which is the most appropriate initial treatment?

A fluid restriction

B intravenous infusion of 0.9% sodium chloride

C rapid intravenous infusion of 3% sodium chloride

D intravenous phenytoin loading

E 2.5 mg bendroflumethiazine (bendrofluazide)

## Question 39

A 56-year-old female presents with thirst and frequency of micturition. These symptoms have deteriorated over the last three months and she is now aware of twice nightly nocturia and occasionally needs to drink during the night. Over this time she has been aware of intermittent frontal headaches, which are generally relieved by paracetamol and are without any relationship to the time of day. She has been rather stressed of late since the breakup of her marriage six months ago. Since the separation she has been taking fluoxetine 20 mg daily. No abnormalities are detected on examination and fasting glucose is 4.2 mmol/L. She undergoes a water deprivation test:

| *Time* | *Weight (kg)* | *Plasma osmolality (mOsmol/kg)* | *Urine osmolality (mOsmol/kg)* | *Urine volume (mL in last hour)* |
|---|---|---|---|---|
| 8 a.m. | 66.5 | 285 | | |
| 9 a.m. | 110 | 200 | | |
| 1 p.m. | 352 | 120 | | |
| 4 p.m. | 65.4 | 303 | 370 | 90 |
| DDVAP 2 μg given intramuscularly at 4pm and patient permitted to drink | | | | |
| 6 p.m. | 66 | 295 | 860 | 20 |

What is the most likely diagnosis?

A central diabetes insipidus

B fluoxetine-induced diabetes insipidus

C nephrogenic diabetes insipidus

D SIADH

E primary polydipsia

## Question 40

A 19-year-old man with severe cognitive impairment was brought to your clinic by his carers. They had noticed that he had been drinking increasing amounts of fluids. His past history included epilepsy, treated with carbamazepine 600 mg twice a day, and asthma.

Fasting blood sugar is normal.

**Further investigations showed:**
plasma osmolality 279 mOsmol/kg (NR 278–305)
urinary osmolality 165 mOsmol/kg (NR 350–1000)

**Eight hours of water-deprivation:**
plasma osmolality 289 mOsmol/kg (NR 278–305)
urinary osmolality 310 mOsmol/kg (NR 350–1000)

**Following 2 μg IM DDAVP:**
plasma osmolality 280 mOsmol/kg (NR 278–305)
urinary osmolality 428 mOsmol/kg (NR 350–1000)

Which of the following is the most likely cause?

A carbamazepine

B compulsive (psychogenic) polydipsia

C cranial diabetes insipidus

D nephrogenic diabetes insipidus

E syndrome of inappropriate antidiuretic hormone (SIADH)

## Question 41

A 40-year-old male is followed up in the renal clinic. His serum creatinine clearance (measured) is 76 mL/min. A recent ultrasound of his renal tract had shown enlarged kidneys bilaterally, with multiple renal cysts. His father required dialysis at the age of 45 years. On examination, his blood pressure is 149/88 mmHg.

Which of the following statements is incorrect in relation to his condition?

A an ACE inhibitor is appropriate to control his hypertension

B he should maintain a high fluid intake

C ciprofloxacin should be prescribed for upper urinary tract infections

D genetic counselling should be offered

E he should be informed of the probable need for dialysis in 5–7 years

## Question 42

A 57-year-old man wishes to act as a kidney donor to his 38-year-old wife. She has end-stage renal failure from polycystic kidney disease and is maintained on peritoneal dialysis. The couple have 12-year-old non-identical twin daughters, neither of whom have renal cysts on recent ultrasound scans.

Which of the following statements is most likely to be correct?

A living-related donation from one of the daughters would be preferable to donation from the husband

B living-unrelated donation is not recommended in cases of inherited renal disease

C the age difference between husband and wife is a relative contraindication to transplantation

D the husband should not be accepted for kidney donation until all siblings have been considered

E the results of living-unrelated kidney donation are sufficiently poor that organ donation should not proceed

## Question 43

Which of the following is **not** a known complication of polycystic kidney disease?

A pancreatic cyst

B mitral valve prolapse

C tricuspid valve incompetence

D subarachnoid haemorrhage

E pulmonary fibrosis

## Question 44

A 48-year-old man with adult polycystic kidney disease who is on maintenance haemodialysis is called for renal transplantation. He had his usual dialysis the previous evening. On examination he has a JVP of +4 cm, BP 140/85 and a clear chest on auscultation. His weight is 2 kg above normal dry weight.

| **Investigations reveal:** | |
|---|---|
| serum sodium | 138 mmol/L |
| serum potassium | 5.5 mmol/L |
| serum bicarbonate | 19 mmol/L |
| **12-lead ECG:** | normal |

The transplant is a good match and surgery is planned for later that day.

What treatment should he receive prior to theatre?

A intravenous fluids

B intravenous insulin + dextrose + salbutamol

C intravenous sodium bicarbonate

D oral calcium resonium

E two hours of haemodialysis

## Question 45

A 20-year-old-male was found by the police in an acutely confused state in the early hours of the morning. He was taken to the local Accident and Emergency Department which, given his history of depression, psychosis and deliberate self-harm, he has attended frequently. He was somewhat agitated with visual hallucinations and a sinus tachycardia (110/min). He told the nursing staff that he had taken some 'acid' of unknown quantity because 'the voice had told him to'. He was observed overnight in hospital and the psychotic symptoms and tachycardia resolved entirely. However, he became frankly depressed. Prior to discharge, his mood improved and he was reviewed by the psychiatric team, who started citalopram. A week later, his mother found him semi-conscious in his flat. His admission electrocardiogram showed a sinus tachycardia of 135/min, his pupils were dilated and he had a temperature of 39.8°C. Blood pressure was 210/105 mmHg. His muscle tone was increased in the legs more than the arms and his reflexes were brisk throughout with equivocal plantars. He was diaphoretic, tremulous and had hyperactive bowel signs.

**Investigations revealed:**

| | |
|---|---|
| haemoglobin | 14.5 g/L |
| white cell count | $8.4 \times 10^9$/L |
| serum sodium | 145 mmol/L |
| serum potassium | 7.3 mmol/L |
| serum urea | 24.3 mmol/L |
| serum creatinine | 610 µmol/L |
| serum bicarbonate | 15 mmol/L |
| **Urinalysis:** | protein (+), blood (+++) |

What is the underlying cause?

A cocaine overdose

B neuroleptic malignant syndrome

C malignant hyperthermia

D serotonin syndrome

E urinary tract infection

## Question 46

A 22-year-old parking attendant for Camden Council, normally fit and well, was referred to hospital by his GP. His only symptoms were of blurred vision and headache that had been present for the preceeding two days. On further questioning the patient also said that he had not been passing much urine and that he had noticed that his breathing had been worse on exertion. There was no history of ankle swelling, but he fell over four days previously and hurt his leg and he had been unable to go out of the house since. There was no history of chest pain.

On examination, he had a regular pulse of 110/minute with a blood pressure of 200/120 mmHg and JVP of 5 cm. His heart sounds were normal. Chest examination revealed fine basal crepitations with a respiratory rate of 22/minute with a sighing pattern. He had boggy tenderness of his right calf and thigh muscles. His abdomen was soft and non-tender with no masses. Fundoscopy was normal. A urinary catheter was then inserted. He was found to have a residual volume of 50 mL of smoky brown urine.

**Investigations revealed:**

**Blood tests:**

| | |
|---|---|
| serum sodium | 135 mmol/L |
| serum potassium | 6.9 mmol/L |
| serum urea | 19.5 mmol/L |
| serum creatinine | 1044 µmol/L |
| serum calcium | 2.0 mmol/L |
| serum phosphate | 2.9 mmol/L |
| serum bicarbonate | 18 mmol/L |
| serum creatine kinase | > 200 iU/L |

**Further tests:**

| | |
|---|---|
| **ECG:** | Sinus tachycardia with no T wave changes |
| **Urinalysis dipstix:** | blood (+++) and protein (++). |
| **Urinary microscopy:** | no organisms, but scanty hyaline casts with fewer than 10 red blood cells per high-powered field. |

What treatment should he receive immediately?

A intravenous 10% calcium chloride

B intravenous 50% dextrose and insulin

C intravenous sodium bicarbonate

D oral calcium resonium

E haemodialysis

# Answers to Chapter 9: Nephrology

These solutions aim to provide the reason(s) for the right answer, and also the reason(s) for the wrong answers being excluded.

1 **Answer C:** Approximately 50% of patients with FSGS do not respond to steroid therapy, but ACE inhibitors are a recognised strategy to slow the progression of renal disease. Having a very high cholesterol, the patient is clearly at high risk of cardiovascular disease, but the question specifically is about renal disease.

2 **Answer D:** The other options cannot explain the findings; in multiple myeloma, one would expect immunoparesis and a paraprotein band; analagesic nephropathy alone would not cause 3.8 g/day proteinuria; acute tubulo-interstitial nephritis is usually associated with haematuria and non-immunogenic amyloidosis is extremely rare and usually presents as familial polyneuropathy.

3 **Answer C:** This lady has longstanding rheumatoid arthritis treated with gold. She currently has an exacerbation of her symptoms. She has renal impairment with mild proteinuria and haematuria. These changes are most suggestive of acute interstitial nephritis, most likely due to NSAID use. NSAIDs may cause renal failure, usually in one of two ways.

Firstly, they inhibit cyclo-oxygenase, which reduces synthesis of the prostaglandins E2 and I2, which are vasodilators that also have a natriuretic effect on the kidney. In individuals with impaired renal perfusion due to, say, hypotension, cirrhosis or cardiac failure, this inhibition may cause a (reversible) fall in GFR, which may then cause acute tubular necrosis and acute renal failure, characterised by fluid retention and hyperkalaemia.

Secondly, NSAIDs may cause an acute allergic interstitial nephritis (AIN), sometimes years after starting the drug. There may be no other clinical features of allergy. Unlike other drugs causing AIN, NSAIDs may cause nephrotic range proteinuria as well as haematuria, white and red cell casts and ARF.

Diagnosis is by renal biopsy.

Treatment is by withdrawal of the causative agent and some nephrologists recommend corticosteroids as they have been shown (anecdotally) to hasten renal recovery. Rarely, NSAIDs may be implicated in vasculitis, glomerulonephritis or renal papillary necrosis. Renal amyloidosis usually presents with nephrotic range proteinuria, renal impairment and normal sized kidneys. Haematuria is rare. Gold use may cause nephrotic syndrome (proteinuria > 3 g/day, oedema and hypoalbuminaemia) and renal biopsy shows membranous nephropathy in 90% of cases. Gold does not usually cause haematuria or ARF. There is no evidence of myeloma in this question. Rheumatoid arthritis may be associated with leucocytoclastic vasculitis which may present with nail-fold infarcts, peripheral neuropathy, pericarditis, GI infarcts or renal failure.

4 **Answer D:** Although hypertension is an early feature of diabetic nephropathy, the diagnostic criteria for diabetes mellitus* have not been met in this patient (HbA1c cannot be used to make a diagnosis of diabetes mellitus). Furthermore, the absence of diabetic retinopathy makes diabetes less likely to be the cause of this patient's renal impairment. The kidneys would be expected to be small, with chronic GN or analgesic nephropathy. Hypertensive nephropathy can present with raised serum creatinine and proteinuria. If the kidneys displayed an asymmetry in size on ultrasound of the renal tract, or if there were a reduction in renal size bilaterally, one would consider renovascular disease.

*Two random glucose measurements of 11.1 mmol/L or more, or two fasting glucose measurements of 7.0 mmol/L or more (one measurement is sufficient if the patient is symptomatic).

5 **Answer C:** Ulcers may be due to large vessel vascular disease, small vessel vascular disease, carcinoma, trauma, or infection. The platelet count was not given. Livedo reticularis results from any disorder impeding drainage of superficial venules to the dermis; therefore, the combination of livedo and ulcers suggests small vessel disease. Endocarditis-induced emboli may produce this, but upper limb signs would be expected and the patient also had negative blood cultures and a normal (transthoracic) echocardiogram.

Cholesterol embolism causes small vessel occlusion and may occur spontaneously, with warfarin or after cardiac catheterisation and should be considered as part of the differential diagnosis of vasculitis in the elderly. The kidneys and lower extremities tend to be preferentially affected. The mechanism of renal damage in cholesterol embolism is not clear but may be due in part to small vessel occlusion by showers of emboli and also to inflammatory cell invasion and subsequent granuloma formation in the vessel wall after the initial ischaemic injury. This may explain the subacute course of the disease. Other clinical features include transient ischaemic attacks, gut haemorrhage or infarction and retinal emboli. Urinalysis may show eosinophiluria. The definitive diagnosis is by renal biopsy and treatment is supportive. Anticoagulation and further arterial instrumentation should be avoided.

6 **Answer C:** The American College of Rheumatology has defined the following criteria for diagnosing SLE:

1 Malar rash
2 Discoid rash
3 Photosensitivity
4 Oral ulcers
5 Arthritis

6 Serositis (pleuritis or pericarditis)
7 Renal disorder (persistent proteinuria or cellular casts)
8 Neurological disorder (seizures or psychosis)
9 Haematological disorder (anemia, leukopenia or lymphopenia on two or more occasions; thrombocytopaenia on one occasion)
10 Immunological disorder (anti-DNA, anti-Sm or antiphospholipid antibodies, false-positive VDRL test)
11 Abnormal antinuclear antibody titre

Four of the above criteria are required (although it is not necessary for all to be present at the same time). In practice, however, SLE is often diagnosed on the basis of typical clinical findings in one organ combined with the presence of circulating autoantibodies.

7 **Answer E:** This man has developed 'pre-renal' renal failure due to sepsis. There is no clear evidence from clinical trials to support the use of any of the above agents, although there is some evidence from animal studies that these agents given early in septicaemia may help prevent renal damage. The use of dopamine, frusemide (furosemide) and mannitol in acute renal failure remains controversial. Treatment should be aimed at optimising cardiovascular status with sufficient fluid (and inotropes if necessary) to maintain blood pressure and end organ perfusion while specific treatment (aimed at the cause of the cardiovascular insufficiency) is given (in this case antibiotics). Renal replacement therapy (dialysis or haemofiltration) is indicated if there is life threatening hyperkalaemia, acidosis, fluid overload or uraemic symptoms (e.g. pericarditis). However, if these conditions do not exist the use of RRT has not been shown to significantly affect speed (or degree) of renal recovery.

8 **Answer A:** Hypovolaemia is by far the most likely cause of his oliguria, and the disproportionally raised serum urea and clear chest x-ray support this. A good response to correction of hypovolaemia would render further investigations unnecessary. Measurement of urine sodium and osmolality and calculation of fractional sodium excretion are used to assess tubular function. In principle, in a hypovolaemic patient with an elevated serum urea and serum creatinine a low urinary sodium (< 20 mmol/L) and high urine osmolality (> 600 mOsmol/kg) represents an appropriate renal response (i.e. retention of salt and water) and is termed 'pre-renal azotemia' in America. If acute tubular necrosis supervenes, this response is lost and urinary sodium loss increases and osmolality decreases. In practice, distinguishing ATN from pre-renal azotemia seldom influences management (which is to correct fluid balance).

9 **Answer B:** The diagnosis is haemolytic uraemic syndrome (HUS), probably caused by *E. coli* serotype 0157:H7. The chief differential diagnosis is between HUS and disseminated intravascular coagulopathy (DIC), but the normal

clotting indices make DIC unlikely. HUS is characterised by MAHA (microangiopathic haemolytic anaemia) with thrombocytopaenia and acute renal failure. MAHA is the result of endothelial damage (in this case by the toxin produced by *E. coli*), leading to adherence of fibrin strands and a rise in von Willebrand multimers, which trap and fragment red cells and platelet count. This produces a characteristic blood picture of anaemia, red cell fragments, thrombocytopaenia and increased reticulocytes. Small vessel fibrin deposition and thrombosis resulting from MAHA lead to renal damage and oliguric renal failure. Treatment of HUS is supportive. Blood transfusions are often necessary. Some 50% of patients require temporary dialysis and 15–40% of patients are left with chronic renal impairment. (*See* **Learning point.**)

10 **Answer E:** The current guidelines issued by the National Kidney Federation are for dialysis patients to have haemoglobin levels maintained at 11 g/dL or more. Blood transfusions should be avoided in dialysis patients, firstly because they have a transient effect on anaemia and secondly to avoid exposure to and immunisation against HLAs, which may complicate subsequent renal transplantation.

A serum ferritin level of less than 80 μg/L in the context of erythrocyte sedimentation rate indicates absolute iron deficiency. A higher serum ferritin does not exclude iron deficiency as serum ferritin is an acute phase protein and may be raised in inflammatory conditions or infections. In this situation, a transferrin saturation of < 20% normally suggests co-existing iron deficiency. Unfortunately, transferrin saturation shows marked diurnal variation and is thus of limited reliability in assessing iron status.

Oral iron supplementation is often poorly tolerated and poorly absorbed by dialysis patients. The response to erythropoietin has been shown to be better with intravenous compared to orally administered iron. This patient is unlikely to respond fully to iron loading as there is a severe normocytic anaemia, so erythropoietin will almost certainly be required.

Other causes of normo- or microcytic anaemia specific to renal dialysis patients include hyperparathyroidism (which is thought to be due to marrow fibrosis) and aluminium toxicity. Aluminium may be used as a phosphate binder or may be found as a contaminant in the water supply for dialysis. Diagnosis is usually by bone biopsy.

11 **Answer C:** Intravenous iron is the first intervention as her percentage of hypochromic red cells is 12% and the high/normal serum ferritin represents an acute phase protein. The goal of iron treatment is usually to maintain the proportion of hyochromic red cells at < 10% and transferrin saturation > 20%. In these conditions, the effect of erythropoietin is maximised.

12 **Answer B:** Amyloidosis is a common cause of musculoskeletal impairment in patients on longstanding dialysis. It is caused by β2 microglobulin

accumulation and causes joint pains and stiffness, often presenting with the classic triad of shoulder pain, carpal tunnel syndrome and flexor tenosynovitis of the hands. Bone cyst formation can lead to pathological fractures (especially of the femoral neck). The only treatment is renal transplantation. It can be reduced by using high flux dialysis membranes in patients who are likely to be on dialysis for a prolonged period.

All of the above options can cause neurological abnormalities in patients with renal failure. Aluminium toxicity can cause twitching, myoclonic jerks, motor apraxia, fits and personality changes (as well as anaemia). It is now rare, due to treatment of dialysis water with reverse osmosis to remove the aluminium, and the use of calcium rather than aluminium containing phosphate binders. The above symptoms do not fit with cerebrovascular disease. Diabetic neuropathy also does not fit with the above picture of symptoms sparing the lower limbs and does not cause stiffness. Uraemia may cause neurological symptoms, more commonly in men, and mostly affecting the legs. Sensory symptoms (paraesthesia, burning sensations and pain) occur before motor symptoms (muscle atrophy, myoclonus, paralysis). The sensory symptoms may improve with starting or increasing the frequency of dialysis, but the motor symptoms are not reversible.

**13 Answer B:** All the clinical details – night sweats, weight loss and spinal pain and tenderness – in combination with antecedent line infection and raised C-reactive protein, suggest ongoing osteomyelitis of the lumbar spine, which is therefore the most likely explanation for his poor responsiveness to erythropoietin. The other options can all cause anaemia unresponsive to erythropoietin but are not suggested by the clinical scenario.

**14 Answer A:** This patient has had a sudden deterioration in renal function, three weeks following an uncomplicated renal transplant. Despite this, she is clinically well, with no symptoms. This lady has acute cellular rejection. Approximately 25% of transplant patients will have at least one episode of rejection, mostly between days 7 and 21, and less commonly up to three months post operation. It is often clinically silent, with only a sharp rise in serum creatinine pointing towards the diagnosis. Doppler ultrasound studies may show a deterioration in graft perfusion, and kidney biopsy will show invading lymphocytes penetrating the tubular basement membrane. Treatment is with high dose steroids. Long-term graft function will be compromised if the rejection episode is not completely reversed.

Symptomatic CMV infection most commonly occurs in the second month after renal transplantation and is usually associated with interstitial pneumonitis, oesophagitis, peptic ulceration, colitis or retinitis. This has been associated with increased graft rejection and renal artery stenosis in renal transplant recipients. In this case there is no suggestion of prodromal active CMV.

Ciclosporin is a calcineurin inhibitor which reduces IL-2 secretion (and therefore T cell proliferation). Like tacrolimus (also a calcineurin inhibitor) ciclosporin is a potent immunosuppressant and is also nephrotoxic. Ciclosporin can cause a dose dependent increase in serum urea and serum creatinine by its vasoconstricting action on the afferent glomerular arteriole (potentiated by NSAIDs). Ciclosporin also may also have a toxic effect on renal tubular cells and can (rarely) cause a haemolytic-uraemic syndrome by its action on endothelial cells. There is no evidence in the question to suggest that the ciclosporin levels are high and the dose has not recently been increased; therefore, this answer is unlikely. The patient is well and there is no suggestion of intercurrent disease causing dehydration. Pyelonephritis of the transplanted kidney is a particular problem in the early immunosuppressed period. It usually presents with low grade pyrexia, tender, swollen graft and deteriorating renal function but may be associated with surprisingly few clinical signs. This lady is well, with no evidence of infection.

15 **Answer A:** This patient has a history of confirmed atherosclerotic coronary artery disease and therefore is at risk of atherosclerosis causing renal artery stenosis. A rise in serum creatinine more than 20% above the baseline after starting an ACEI should prompt the clinician to stop the drug, monitor renal function and consider renal imaging. The patient does not have diabetes, based on a fasting plasma glucose of only 6 mmol/L.

Angiotensin II is a vasoconstricting hormone which affects the renal efferent arteriole more potently than the afferent. This maintains the pressure across the glomerular basement membrane in the presence of renal hypoperfusion (due, for instance, to systemic hypotension or renal artery stenosis). If renal perfusion is sufficiently impaired then the glomerular filtration rate is critically dependent on this effect, and drugs which block the renin-angiotensin axis can cause a significant enough reduction in GFR to cause renal failure. This usually reverses on stopping the causative drug.

The treatment of RAS is usually by control of hypertension (and other cardiovascular risk factors). Randomised controlled trials of renal artery angioplasty and medical therapy in atherosclerotic renal artery stenosis have not consistently shown that angioplasty significantly improves either blood pressure control or renal function. However, some nephrologists hold the view that angioplasty may delay progression of renal impairment.

16 **Answer E:** This patient has renal impairment and cardiovascular disease. Serum creatinine rose following the administration of an angiotensin converting enzyme inhibitor (ACE-I) and renovascular disease is the most likely explanation. Her renal impairment should improve on cessation of ACEI and the electrolytes will then normalise.

If she had marked hyperkalaemia with ECG changes then haemodialysis would possibly be required. Sodium bicarbonate infusion is reasonable if there is severe hyperkalaemia and acidosis, as raising the serum pH can cause an intracellular shift of potassium. However, sodium loading a patient who has myocardial ischaemia may cause fluid overload and pulmonary oedema. Insulin and dextrose infusion will result in a temporary shift of potassium from the vascular compartment into cells which may last a few hours at the most. Calcium resonium may ameliorate hyperkalaemia over the course of 6–12 hours, but it does not address the cause of worsening renal function. It should be used as a temporary measure to lower serum potassium while awaiting dialysis or if significant improvement in renal function is expected.

Peripherally infused concentrated salts (e.g. 10% calcium chloride or 8.4% sodium bicarbonate) carry a significant risk of severe tissue injury (which may require skin grafting) if they extravasate. Their use should therefore be reserved for patients with ECG changes of hyperkalaemia in whom rapid treatment is necessary to prevent cardiac arrest.

**17** **Answer C:** The constellation of asthma, eosinophilia, mononeuritis multiplex, detectable ANCA and acute renal failure suggests Churg-Strauss syndrome, which is a small to medium-sized vasculitis that also has a predilection for the bowel. Presentation may be with pulmonary haemorrhage and renal involvement is less common than in Wegener's granulomatosis. The renal lesion in Churg-Strauss syndrome is usually a focal necrotising glomerulonephritis but in some cases biopsy reveals a florid interstitial nephritis with eosinophil invasion. Treatment is with steroids, but in severe cases further immunosuppression is required. Response to treatment is usually good, with remission rates being > 90%. The major cause of ongoing morbidity is from the mononeuritis multiplex.

**18** **Answer A:** This lady probably has Henoch-Schonlein purpura (HSP). A renal biopsy would show mesangial and capillary wall IgA staining and mesangial electron dense deposits on electron microscopy. This is an identical picture to that seen in IgA nephropathy and the two conditions are differentiated only by the presence of extra-renal features in HSP.

IgA nephropathy and HSP often present 1–3 days following infection of an IgA-secreting mucous membrane (commonly pharyngitis, but they can also occur following infection of the GI tract, bladder or breast). This contrasts with post-infectious (or post-streptococcal) GN where there is a delay of 10–14 days between onset of infection and renal symptoms. The renal presentation in IgA nephropathy is usually with painless macroscopic haematuria and proteinuria, or less commonly nephrotic syndrome (approximately 5%) or microscopic haematuria. The rash in HSP is due to a cutaneous vasculitis, and the abdominal pain is due to gut vasculitis, which may lead to intussusception and bloody diarrhoea. Arthralgia is a common symptom.

The presence of significant proteinuria (> 1g/day) is a risk factor for the development of end stage renal failure. Patients with hypertension and proteinuria (> 1g/day – which this patient probably has) should be started on an ACE inhibitor, which may control the BP and proteinuria.

The evidence for immunosuppressive therapy in IgA/HSP is poor and it is usually reserved for patients with acute renal failure and significant proteinuria, nephrotic syndrome or diffuse crescentic glomerulonephritis on renal biopsy. (*See* **Learning point**.)

**19 Answer E.**

**20 Answer B:** Reflux nephropathy is the most likely underlying diagnosis.

Vesicoureteric reflux (VUR), which is the retrograde flow of urine from the bladder up into the ureters, is often found in children with recurrent urinary tract infections. At presentation or subsequently, a small proportion of such children are found to have a characteristic pattern of renal parenchymal scarring at the upper and lower poles, with underlying clubbing and distortion of calyces. This pattern of scarring is termed reflux nephropathy (or chronic pyelonephritis). These patients have an increased risk of recurrent urinary tract infection and may develop proteinuria, renal stones, hypertension and progressive renal impairment, with an inexorable progression to endstage renal failure. This may occur even if the underlying defect (vesicoureteric reflux) resolves, as it often does as the child gets older.

The diagnosis of reflux nephropathy is best made in adults by intravenous urography which shows focal parenchymal scarring and calyceal abnormalities. Ultrasound may show focal scarring but does not allow visualisation of the calyces. In children (in whom there are few alternative causes of focal scarring) DMSA isotope scanning is a more sensitive test and isotope micturating cystourography may demonstrate vesicoureteric reflux, confirming the diagnosis. This test is rarely used in adults, as reflux often resolves with age and its presence will not alter management.

**21 Answer E:** This lady is probably experiencing abdominal discomfort because of recurrent urinary tract infections. The small kidney on the right hand side is a consequence of renal scarring due to vesicoureteric reflux and recurrent urinary tract infections earlier in life.

Vesicoureteric reflux is found in 5–20% of young children with urinary tract infection, is the commonest cause of childhood hypertension and may lead to chronic renal failure. VUR may occur either due to bladder outflow obstruction or as a primary developmental abnormality at the vesicoureteric junction. The diagnosis is usually made by voiding cystourethrography in childhood, which also allows the severity of reflux to be graded. Renal damage is thought to be due to reflux of infected urine into the collecting system, so management is based around early treatment and prophylaxis of urinary tract infections as well as hypertension. VUR tends to resolve by adulthood. However, any renal scarring remains and may lead to CRF in adulthood. The diagnosis in adults is usually made by ultrasound or by intravenous urography, which may show evidence of loss of renal substance, focal scarring at the renal poles or dilated (or 'clubbed') pelvi-calyceal systems.

Renal asymmetry is unlikely with chronic glomerulonephritis or IgA nephropathy. With fibromuscular dysplasia, there might be evidence of more significant hypertension, and possibly end organ disease. Congenital renal atrophy would not cause abdominal pain or urine dipstick abnormalities.

22 **Answer E:** This man has had a calcium urinary tract stone. He has normal serum calcium but raised urinary excretion of calcium. Idiopathic hypercalciuria is often familial, the most common cause being increased gastrointestinal absorption of calcium. Further investigation may reveal a raised vitamin D level or, more rarely, raised bone turnover and reduced bone density.

Approximately 65–80% of renal stones contain calcium oxalate. These are five times more common in males due to testosterone's effect on hepatic glycolic acid oxidase activity. Up to 40% of urinary oxalate is derived from dietary ascorbic acid. Normally only 5% of dietary oxalate is absorbed, but if dietary calcium is restricted, oxalate absorption may increase to 10%. Preventing calcium oxalate stones therefore depends on maintaining sufficient urine flow (2 litres per day) to minimise stone formation. Thiazide diuretics reduce renal tubular calcium excretion, and therefore can prevent calcium stone formation. Loop diuretics increase urinary excretion of calcium, and therefore would exacerbate calcium renal stone formation.

A high dietary protein intake is associated with urinary stones, and oxalate-containing foods should be avoided. There is no evidence that dietary restriction of calcium intake is of value, as any benefit would be offset by increased oxalate absorption.

Natural inhibitors (most importantly citrate) prevent crystal nucleation in supersaturated urine. Hypocitraturia may be a consequence of systemic acidosis, hypokalaemia and hypomagnesaemia. Oral citrate supplementation has not been shown to be of benefit unless there is hypocitraturia.

Struvite stones account for approximately 20% of renal stones and are usually a consequence of urease-producing organisms (e.g. *Proteus*) chronically infecting the urinary tract. They occur in 5–10% of people with spinal cord injury and up to 30% of people with ileal conduits and may form staghorn calculi requiring surgical treatment.

Other types of renal stone, such as urate (7%), cystine (1%) and xanthine (< 1%), are rare.

Allopurinol would reduce the incidence of uric acid stones and potassium bicarbonate can be used to alkalinise the urine, reducing the formation of most stones. These agents have no significant effect on the formation of calcium-containing stones in idiopathic hypercalciuric stone-formers.

23 **Answer C:** In small bowel disease, fat malabsorption causes calcium-fat complexes (saponification) in the intestine, reducing calcium-oxalate complexes. This leads to raised oxalate absorption and hyperoxaluria, which may then cause stone formation. It is important to note that this patient will be more susceptible to all forms of stone disease, as inflammatory bowel disease predisposes to dehydration (low urine volume) and reduced urinary crystal inhibitors (e.g. citrate, magnesium and phosphate).

24 **Answer B:** Since this patient already drinks 3 litres of fluid per day, further increase in fluid intake is unlikely to be as beneficial as reducing consumption of oxalate. Low-oxalate diets typically exclude cocoa, peanut products, rhubarb, beetroot, spinach, tofu and soya beans.

25 **Answer B:** The combination of retinopathy, significant microalbuminuria and very poor glycaemic control requires aggressive treatment to minimise end-organ damage (i.e. renal failure and blindness). The Diabetic Control and Complications Trial (*NEJM* 1993) demonstrated a significant reduction in retinopathy, micro- and macroalbuminuria and neuropathy, with tighter glycaemic control in people with type 1 diabetes. The chief adverse event was a two- to three-fold increase in severe hypoglycaemic attacks.

The role of ACE inhibitors in normotensive diabetic patients with micro- and macroalbuminuria is well established, also by randomised controlled trials, and these patients should all receive these agents if tolerated. It is also important to control any hyperlipidaemia, as this is associated with more rapid progression once nephropathy is established.

26 **Answer E:** Fatigue and weight loss are symptoms of insulin deficiency. These, combined with evidence of poor glycaemic control (raised HbA1C) and established retinopathy and nephropathy are indications for starting insulin therapy. Most authorities recommended that metformin should be stopped in patients with a serum creatinine above 150 µmol/L due to the risk of severe, life-threatening lactic acidosis. Although rosiglitazone could be added to existing oral hypoglycaemic agents, it is unlikely to provide much benefit in this patient.

Glibenclamide should also be avoided in renal failure due to its long duration of action and risk of hypoglycaemia. Gliclazide, which is metabolised by the liver, is a better choice of oral hypoglycaemic therapy in renal failure.

27 **Answer D:** Strict glycaemic control would reduce the frequency of recurrent infections and reduce the risk of progression to diabetic nephropathy. If she had proteinuria in the absence of proven UTI, she would also benefit from an ACE inhibitor, regardless of the blood pressure. However, this would not decrease the frequency of UTIs. Stopping smoking would be beneficial in reducing the risk of developing future vascular disease. Prophylactic antibiotics are of benefit in preserving renal function with recurrent UTIs, and should

be offered if the patient is symptomatic with her infections. Vesicoureteric reflux usually occurs early in childhood, and it is at this juncture that any surgical intervention would be beneficial. When picked up in adulthood, the mainstay of management would be blood pressure control, prompt treatment of UTI and careful surveillance during pregnancy.

**28** **Answer B:** This patient appears to have an established nephropathy, with (++) protein on urinalysis and poor hypertensive control. The most likely underlying diagnosis is diabetic renal disease and the best antihypertensive agent is likely to be an ACE inhibitor. It may be that further antihypertensives (e.g. a thiazide diuretic, a beta blocker or an alpha blocker) are needed to keep the blood pressure below target. Further investigation to exclude renal artery stenosis (i.e. renal vessel MRA) would be indicated if there were asymmetry in renal size on ultrasound or if the renal function deteriorated significantly (serum creatinine rise of 15%) after starting an ACE inhibitor.

Metformin should not be used with this degree of renal impairment, due to the risk of life-threatening lactic acidosis. Glibenclamide is also a poor choice of oral hypoglycaemic agent in renal failure as it is long-acting and renally excreted. It is likely that this man requires insulin therapy to maintain adequate glycaemic control.

He would require further investigation of the blood and protein in the urine, but in the first instance the patient needs urgent control of his blood pressure. Target BP for patients with type 2 diabetes and any other cardiovascular risk factors (e.g. microalbuminuria or renal disease) is < 140/80, as described in the NICE guidelines.

**29** **Answer B:** At 13 weeks of pregnancy, it is too early to present with pre-eclampsia (which should only be diagnosed after 20 weeks). Fibromuscular dysplasia causing renal artery stenosis does not typically present with dipstick haematuria. Membranous GN is associated with nephrotic syndrome and therefore one would expect more proteinuria and no haematuria. This patient has normal sized kidneys, which would be unusual for reflux nephropathy. IgA nephropathy can present with all the above features.

**30** **Answer C:** The microcytic anaemia and African origin suggest an underlying diagnosis of sickle cell disease in this patient. In this context, painless macroscopic haematuria is most likely to be due to an ischaemic lesion of the renal papilla, causing papillary necrosis. Treatment is conservative, although prolonged haematuria may require transfusion or limited surgery.

There is nothing in the question to point to a diagnosis of analgesic nephropathy. Renal vein thrombosis may be associated with flank pain and should be suspected in haematuria if there is nephrotic syndrome or another cause of hypercoagulability. The absence of a systemic inflammatory response argues against malaria or pyelonephritis.

31 **Answer B:** There is a well recognised association of Hodgkin's Disease with minimal change glomerulonephropathy. Heavy metal poisoning tends to cause renal tubular damage and penicillamine is associated with membranous nephropathy. Many other factors (e.g. allergies and EBV infection) have been implicated in minimal change disease but a causative role has not been proven.

32 **Answer E:** This gentleman has nephrotic syndrome and evidence of renal impairment that improves markedly with oral prednisolone. This is highly suggestive of minimal change disease, in which up to 80% of adult patients respond well to steroids alone.

Antiglomerular basement membrane disease causes a rapidly progressive glomerulonephritis which may be associated with pulmonary haemorrhage (in which case it is termed Goodpasture's disease), which requires treatment with high dose intravenous methylprednisolone and cyclophosphamide. It would not improve with oral prednisolone alone. Plasma exchange is indicated if there is pulmonary haemorrhage or if the patient is dialysis dependent at presentation.

IgA disease rarely causes nephrotic syndrome (approximately 5% of cases). High dose prednisolone can be used in patients with nephrotic range proteinuria in IgA nephropathy, but the improvement seen in the question would be unusual.

In patients with membranous glomerulonephritis, there is no clear agreement about the best treatment. However, most authorities agree that steroid therapy alone is unlikely to be of benefit. High dose cytotoxic therapy (the Ponticelli regime) has had good results in randomised controlled trials in Italy. Heavy proteinuria and renal failure at presentation are predictors of poor prognosis.

Progression of mesangiocapillary glomerulonephritis may be slowed by treatment with antiplatelet drugs, anticoagulants, corticosteroids and alkylating agents. Steroids are given for a prolonged period of time, and evidence suggests they are of some benefit. In this question, the dramatic response seen to steroids alone would be highly unusual in mesangiocapillary glomerulonephritis.

33 **Answer A:** Membranous glomerulonephritis is one of the commonest causes of nephrotic syndrome in adults in the UK. It can occur as a primary disorder or secondary to a wide range of systemic disease including hepatitis B, malaria, malignancy, sarcoidosis, autoimmune disorders (e.g. SLE) and drugs (e.g. penicillamine and gold). Renal biopsy shows thickening of the glomerular basement membrane with IgG and C3 on immunostaining.

The clinical course is variable and difficult to predict. Remission can occur after years of nephrotic range proteinuria, and renal function may decline and then improve. Progression to end stage renal failure occurs in up to 20% and may be reduced by cytotoxic therapy.

**34** **Answer D:** This patient has a relapse of her nephrotic syndrome, causing oedema, hypoalbuminaemia and hypercoagulability. The lack of response to heparin is almost certainly due to (acquired) antithrombin III deficiency. Heparin acts primarily by potentiating the action of antithrombin III, the concentration of which can fall as low as 10–20% of normal (through urinary loss) in patients with nephrotic syndrome.

Various coagulation factors (both pro- and anti-coagulant) are lost in the urine in the nephrotic syndrome, but some more than others, and the net effect is usually to produce a procoagulant state. The plasma concentration of protein C is usually normal in nephrotic syndrome (despite some urinary losses).

There is no evidence in this question that the patient had a pre-existing procoagulant state (e.g. the inherited factor V Leiden mutation or inherited protein C deficiency) and the antiphospholipid syndrome would be expected to cause an artificially raised APTT ratio and a procoagulant state. Antiphospholipid syndrome is not usually caused by minimal change glomerulonephritis. Most nephrologists would treat this patient with warfarin.

**35** **Answer D:** This female patient has weight gain, abdominal swelling and ankle oedema associated with hypertension, mild anaemia and proteinuria. It would be vital to exclude pregnancy and associated pre-eclampsia with a urinary BhCG test before undertaking further investigations.

**36** **Answer D:** This patient has the nephrotic syndrome as defined by a triad of hypoalbuminaemia, proteinuria > 3 g/24hrs and oedema. The commonest cause of nephrotic syndrome in a child is minimal change disease, which usually responds to a course of high dose corticosteroids. Cyclophosphamide may hasten a remission but, given its cytotoxic profile and significant risk of infertility, should be reserved for steroid-resistant cases and, if possible, should be avoided entirely in childhood. Salt-poor serum albumin and intravenous frusemide (furosemide) may be useful adjuncts for managing oedema, but in this patient steroids are likely to be more effective. If the nephrotic syndrome is left unchecked, complications include overwhelming streptococcal sepsis, venous thromboembolism and hypercholesterolaemia. Renal failure in the nephrotic syndrome can be caused by progression of underlying glomerular disorder, hypovolaemia (due to over-diuresis for oedema), renal vein thrombosis or sepsis. ARF is rare in childhood nephrotic syndrome.

**37** **Answer E:** The differential diagnosis in the postoperative neurosurgical patient with hyponatraemia is usually between SIADH and cerebral salt wasting, both of which commonly occur in these patients. In this question, the postural drop, tachycardia and rising serum urea suggest that the patient is dehydrated and the urine output is inappropriately high (averaging 160 mL/h) and contains large quantities of sodium. This is highly suggestive of a salt wasting state.

Cerebral salt wasting was first described in 1950 and is thought by some to be at least as common as SIADH in neurosurgical patients. The pathophysiology is poorly understood but it is thought that inappropriate release of natriuretic peptides following cerebral injury may play a role.

In SIADH, one would expect to see a euvolaemic patient with a relatively low urine output. The urine would be hypertonic but total sodium excretion would be similar to intake. Serum urate is usually low.

It is important to differentiate these two conditions as the treatment for one is completely inappropriate for the other. The patient in this question should receive fluid to correct the hypovolaemia and sodium to replace the excessive loss. In SIADH, the defect is impaired free water excretion and any fluid given would exacerbate the hyponatraemia. Sodium supplementation would be ineffective for SIADH as it would be excreted by the kidneys.

Cranial diabetes insipidus also may occur following neurosurgery or head injuries, but causes hypernatraemia due to the production of inappropriately dilute urine. Hypoadrenalism, like hypothyroidism, may cause hyponatraemia but is less likely in this situation. These two treatable endocrine conditions should be excluded in all hyponatraemic patients.

**38** **Answer C:** The diagnosis here is syndrome of inappropriate ADH, probably secondary to the lung neoplasm. The diagnosis is confirmed by the euvolaemic state, hyponatraemia and inappropriately concentrated urine. SIADH will respond to fluid restriction; however, this patient has clear evidence of neurological consequences of severe hyponatraemia and therefore this warrants *rapid* correction. Cranial CT imaging would also be needed in this patient to exclude cerebral metastases.

It is important to recognise that symptomatic hyponatraemia requires rapid correction, notwithstanding the risk of central pontine myelinolysis, because seizures carry a definite morbidity and mortality in themselves whereas CPM is a theoretical risk. Once the neurological symptoms have stopped, the sodium should be brought up slowly (by not more than 10 mmol/L per day).

Fluid restriction is effective in SIADH but usually brings the sodium up slowly, which is ideal in asymptomatic patients, but not in those having seizures.

0.9% sodium chloride solution may worsen hyponatraemia in SIADH because the sodium content will be excreted by the kidneys but the water is retained, decreasing serum sodium.

Antiepileptic drugs are unlikely to be effective in seizures caused by hyponatraemia (the antiepileptic drugs carbamazepine and oxcarbazepine commonly cause or exacerbate hyponatraemia).

Although loop diuretics may be of benefit in SIADH, thiazides cause a natriuresis by blocking sodium resorption in the early distal tubule and will therefore *worsen* hyponatraemia. (*See* **Learning point.**)

39 **Answer A:** This patient has developed haemoconcentration following eight hours of dehydration. Although there is slight concentration of her urine this is inadequate to maintain plasma osmolality and the urine output is still high, eight hours into the test. The fact that she has lost weight over the first eight hours of the test demonstrates that there was no surreptitious drinking. There is a good response to DDAVP, indicating that she has central rather than nephrogenic diabetes insipidus.

Fluoxetine does not cause DI but may cause SIADH.

40 **Answer B:** This patient has a low normal plasma osmolality and low urine osmolality, both of which increase during the water deprivation test. Compulsive polydipsia fits with this pattern of findings. His urine starts to concentrate during the water deprivation test but there is only a small change in serum osmolality (which is maintained within the normal range). These patients are best managed by stopping fluid replacement and asking the patient to drink only when thirsty. Paired urine and serum osmolalities should then be conducted at regular intervals to ensure that the osmolalities are returning to normal. The changes in his plasma and urine osmolalities following the test are not large. This is because prolonged polyuria leads to a reduction in the maximal concentrating ability of the kidney by removing renal medullary interstitial solute. DDAVP (a synthetic vasopressin analogue) is therefore unable to elicit its maximal effect of increasing water reabsorption. Cranial diabetes insipidus (DI) is caused by decreased secretion of vasopressin from the posterior pituitary. In cranial DI the plasma osmolality following the water deprivation test would rise, and an effect would be seen following administration of desmopressin (increased urine osmolality). Nephrogenic diabetes insipidus is caused by renal tubular resistance to vasopressin and therefore the plasma osmolality would rise during the water deprivation test, but the urine would remain dilute, even after desmopressin administration.

Carbamazepine causes a syndrome of inappropriate ADH. This would be associated with concentrated urine (high osmolality), and dilute serum (low osmolality). The urine osmolality would not change during the water deprivation test.

41 **Answer E:** This patient has autosomal dominant polycystic kidney disease (ADPKD or PKD). 75% of patients progress to end-stage renal failure between the ages of 50 and 75 (only 15% require dialysis below the age of 50). Renal function usually deteriorates in a gradual fashion, with a drop in serum creatinine clearance of approximately 5 mL/min/year. Treatment should include a high fluid intake (to prevent the formation of renal stones

or blood clots) and regular follow-up of blood pressure and renal function. Loin pain should be treated symptomatically, and hypertension should be managed with standard anti-hypertensive medications. Haematuria should be treated conservatively. Urinary tract infections should be treated with lipophillic drugs (e.g. ciprofloxacin, trimethoprim or metronidazole) as they have better penetration into cyst fluid than non-lipophilic antibiotics (such as aminoglycosides and cephalosporins). As an autosomal dominant disease, APKD gives the offspring of an affected patient a 50% chance of inheriting the condition. The patient should be offered genetic counselling, despite the fact that the disease has a variable clinical course even between affected family members.

42 **Answer D:** Provided that there is a sibling who is proven not to have polycystic kidney disease, living-related donation should be considered as there would probably be a better HLA match and therefore better graft survival. Living-unrelated kidney donation produces excellent results (regardless of HLA haplotype) compared to cadaveric renal transplants, even if the latter are well-matched. In patients with polycystic kidney disease, a graft from an unrelated donor would not succumb to the same disease process. Provided the donor is fit and well (with good renal function), the age difference would not be considered a contraindication to kidney donation.

In the UK currently, live kidney donation is only allowed between people who can demonstrate an 'emotional' relationship – usually spouses and 1st degree relatives. Many people decline to accept kidneys from their children, and 12 years old is usually considered too young to exclude autosomal dominant polycystic kidney disease by ultrasound scanning.

43 **Answer E:** All of the other options are associated with autosomal dominant polycystic kidney disease. Other associations include cysts of the liver, spleen, ovary, and also hernias of the anterior abdominal wall. Aortic valve prolapse also has an increased incidence in patients with ADPKD.

Intracranial (berry) aneurysms are found in approximately 8% of asymptomatic patients with ADPKD (compared to 1.2% of the general UK population), so people with ADPKD have a correspondingly greater incidence of subarachnoid haemorrhage. Screening with magnetic resonance angiography should be considered in patients with ADPKD aged between 18–35 who have a family history of intracranial aneurysm.

44 **Answer E:** Haemodialysis will correct his fluid, acid base and electrolyte balance.

45 **Answer D:** The combination of tremor, increased muscle tone, brisk reflexes, mydriasis, diaphoresis, hypertension and hyperthermia is diagnostic of the serotonin syndrome in a person exposed to a serotoninergic drug. These include selective serotonin reuptake inhibitors (e.g. citalopram), other

antidepressants, monoamine oxidase inhibitors, certain opioid analgesics, sumatriptan, lithium, ecstasy, and LSD. Untreated, the serotonin syndrome may cause rhabdomyolysis and consequent acute renal failure. Treatment is initially with fluids, withdrawal of serotoninergic agents and benzodiazepines for agitation. The 5-HT2A receptor antagonist cyproheptadine can be used for more severe cases.

Neuroleptic malignant syndrome causes bradyreflexia, decreased bowel sounds and lead-pipe rigidity and does not cause mydriasis. It is also associated with hyperpyrexia and rhabdomyolysis. Malignant hyperthermia may occur after administration of an inhalational anaesthetic and causes hyporeflexia, decreased bowel sounds and no pupil abnormalities. It can also lead to rhabdomyolysis.

**46 Answer B:** Rhabdomyolysis features regularly in the MRCP examination, and can be due to a number of medical disorders. This man has rhabdomyolysis, and therefore the immediate treatment is correction of his potassium, fluid balance and acidosis. (*See* **Learning point.**)

Intravenous insulin and dextrose is the best option, immediately followed by aggressive rehydration and careful monitoring of fluid balance, acidosis and serum potassium (usually with a CVP line). Thereafter if urine output cannot be maintained or if potassium remains elevated, dialysis may be necessary. Severe rebound hypercalcaemia is sometimes seen in the recovery phase and is thought to be due to secondary (appropriate) hyperparathyroidism. This complication can be prevented to some degree by avoiding calcium therapy during the acute stage. However, symptomatic hypocalcaemia should not be left untreated, especially if there is coexisting hyperkalaemia due to the risk of cardiac arrest.

In the absence of either extreme hyperkalaemia (> 7.5 mmol/L) or ECG changes suggesting impending cardiac dysfunction or arrest, peripheral administration of concentrated salts (e.g. calcium chloride or sodium bicarbonate) should be avoided.

# Learning Points

## *Question 9*

### Learning point

**Causes of MAHA**

HUS

Thrombotic thrombocytopaenic purpura

Obstetric complications (HELLP syndrome, amniotic fluid embolism, septic abortion)

Accelerated hypertension

Septicaemia/DIC

Vasculitides

Metastatic carcinoma

Burns

Prosthetic valve-induced haemolysis

Drugs (ciclosporin, tacrolimus, mitomycin C)

## *Question 18*

### Learning point

**Microscopic haematuria**

Microscopic haematuria has many renal and urological (e.g. urothelial cancer, prostatic disease, stones) causes, but the presence of red cell casts, significant proteinuria, hypertension and renal impairment suggests glomerulonephritis. The commonest glomerular causes of microscopic haematuria are:

- IgA nephropathy: patients often have episodes of macroscopic haematuria concurrent with upper respiratory tract infection. Most cases of IgA nephropathy are idiopathic, but this type of glomerulonephritis is also commonly associated with Henoch-Schonlein purpura and alcoholic cirrhosis. Biopsy shows diffuse mesangial deposits of IgA.

- Thin basement-membrane disease: a familial disorder which presents with isolated microscopic haematuria, minimal proteinuria and normal renal function which does not deteriorate. Electron microscopy shows diffuse thinning of the glomerular basement membrane (the width is usually between 150 and 225 nM versus 300–400 nM in normal subjects).
- Alport's disease: this is a progressive form of glomerular disease, associated with deafness and ocular abnormalities and is usually inherited as an X-linked dominant condition (although males are more seriously affected than females).

Other renal disorders which should be considered in the differential diagnosis of microscopic haematuria include polycystic kidney disease, renal papillary necrosis, loin pain haematuria syndrome, renal vein thrombosis, sickle-cell disease and schistosomiasis.

## *Question 38*

### Learning point

**Causes of SIADH**

Drugs: chlorpropamide, chlorpromazine, carbamazepine, oxcarbazepine, opiates, vincristine.

Central nervous system: head injury, encephalitis/meningitis, cerebral abscess, cerebral neoplasm, cerebral haemorrhage

Respiratory system: bronchial carcinoma (particularly small cell), tuberculosis, pneumonia (*Legionnaire's disease appears to be the College's examination favourite!*), empyema

Miscellaneous: Guillain-Barré syndrome, acute intermittent porphyria, carcinoma of the pancreas/thymoma.

## *Question 45*

### Learning point

**Causes of rhabdomyolysis**

Trauma (compartment syndrome, bullet wounds, road traffic accidents); prolonged epileptic seizures; alcohol excess; temperature excess (malignant hyperthermia or environmental), drug intoxication (cocaine and Ecstasy, or prolonged immobility from any other cause), hereditary (e.g. McArdle's syndrome).

# CHAPTER 10

# Neurology, ophthalmology and psychiatry

Neurology, ophthalmology and psychiatry tend to be areas people dread the most. Questions here are supposed to test your knowledge of common disorders of clinical neurology, psychiatry and ophthalmology. The choice of subjects will include the common emergencies usually, and topics which have attracted recent attention, such as the management of transient ischaemic attacks and stroke.

## CEREBROSPINAL FLUID

| | |
|---|---|
| opening pressure | 50–180 mm $H_2O$ |
| total protein | 0.15–0.45 g/L |
| serum albumin | 0.066–0.442 g/L |
| chloride | 116–122 mmol/L |
| glucose | 3.3–4.4 mmol/L |
| lactate | 1 –2 mmol/L |
| cell count | ≤ 5 $mL^{-1}$ |

# Questions

## Question 1

A 59-year-old man, recently retired from a lifelong career in the civil service, was brought to see his GP by his wife, who had noticed that he often had histories of forgetting. Due to having time to pursue his hobbies, he himself reported that his mood was quite good. His wife, in private, reported him as being rather impulsive while shopping with his credit card. He had also acquired a marked taste for sweet foods and fizzy drinks (unusual for him). His memory for both recent and past events was excellent. Clinical examination was normal, and his bedside score on the MMSE was 29 (out of 30). His uncle had died of pneumonia, after a long illness of Parkinson's disease. The GP started him on a course of anti-depressants, which had no effect.

What is the most likely diagnosis?

A Alzheimer's disease

B depression

C familial Parkinson's disease

D frontotemporal degeneration

E old age

## Question 2

A 45-year-old man with a medical history of multiple sclerosis was admitted to hospital following an overdose of baclofen. He was diagnosed with relapsing and remitting multiple sclerosis 20 years ago and is usually mobile with two sticks. He performs intermittent self-catheterisation and his only medication is baclofen 20 mg three times a day. He was found by his son surrounded by empty baclofen packets after returning from a night out with his friends. Earlier that evening, the patient and his partner had had an argument and this was thought to have precipitated his actions. According to his partner, there had been approximately twenty tablets left in the packet, each containing 10 mg of baclofen (150 mg of baclofen is associated with severe toxicity). He is a non-smoker and is teetotal. The only other medical history of note is a previous admission 18 months ago with severe community acquired pneumonia, for which he needed mechanical ventilation. On examination, he was drowsy with a respiratory rate of five breaths per minute. He had a Glasgow Coma Scale (GCS) of 8/15, and a neurological examination revealed generalised hyporeflexia. The pulse was 60/min and regular, and blood pressure was 96/60. Examination of respiratory, cardiovascular and abdominal system was unremarkable.

His arterial gases (on 50% inspired $O_2$) were as follows:

| | |
|---|---|
| pH | 7.34 |
| $pO_2$ | 24 kPa |
| $pCO_2$ | 7.2 kPa |
| $HCO_3$ | 27 mmol/L |
| base excess | 0.3 |

What is an appropriate next step in this patient's management?

A increased concentration of inspired oxygen

B intravenous doxapram infusion

C intubation and mechanical ventilation

D non-invasive positive pressure ventilation (NIPPV)

E reduce concentration of inspired oxygen

## Question 3

A 68-year-old lady presents with painful arms. She is noted to be dyspnoeic and tachypnoeic at rest, and both clinical examination and chest film reveal a right-sided pleural effusion. She has a mild proximal myopathy. The Casualty officer requests a 'routine' blood analysis:

**Investigations reveal:**

**Blood tests:**

| | |
|---|---|
| serum creatinine kinase | 425 U/L |
| haemoglobin | 10.8 g/L |
| white cell count | $7.9 \times 10^9$/L |
| platelet count | $190 \times 10^9$/L |
| **Blood film:** | anisocytosis, with mild macrocytosis |

The most likely diagnosis is:

A rhabdomyolysis

B polymyositis

C muscular dystrophy

D hypothyroidism

E dermatomyositis

## Question 4

An 80-year-old man, previously fit and healthy, presents with severe flinging movements of the left arm.

Where is the neurological lesion?

A caudate nucleus

B globus pallidus

C ipsilateral thalamus

D substantia nigra

E subthalamic nucleus

## Question 5

A 29-year-old news presenter from Pimlico attended Outpatient clinic after a positive pregnancy test. She was diagnosed with epilepsy at the age of 19, having suffered two tonic-clonic seizures. At the time of diagnosis, she was started on sodium valproate. She took this subsequently without any further seizure. She last had a period 13 weeks previously, having usually had a regular 28 day menstrual cycle.

What decision is most appropriate regarding her anticonvulsant therapy?

A continue sodium valproate

B convert sodium valproate to carbamazepine

C convert sodium valproate to lamotrigine

D reduce the dose of sodium valproate

E stop anticonvulsant therapy

## Question 6

A 23-year-old woman presents to her GP complaining of impaired sweating in hot weather. She feels that the onset of her symptoms was sudden, and on examination she has a sluggishly reactive pupil. The only other physical sign is absent ankle jerks, even with reinforcement. She otherwise feels well.

The nature of the pathology is best described as:

A Holmes-Adie pupil

B ptosis

C Horner's syndrome

D Argyll-Robinson pupil

E third nerve palsy

## Question 7

A 60-year-old woman presented with a small right pupil, right sided ptosis, and impaired sweating over the ipsilateral forehead. Sweating on the rest of the face was unaffected.

The most likely site of the lesion is:

A cervical spinal cord

B common carotid artery

C hypothalamus

D internal carotid artery

E lateral medulla

## Question 8

A 36-year-old presents with severe unsteadiness, difficulty in swallowing, and intractable hiccups, accompanied by nausea, deafness, and vomiting. On examination, he has marked limb ataxia, impairment of sensation on the left side of his face, impairment of left sided eye abduction, a left facial nerve palsy, and a mild left-sided Horner's syndrome. He has loss of contalateral pain and temperature sensation. Cerebellar signs are elicited on the left.

The vessel most likely to be occluded is:

A left posterior inferior cerebellar artery

B right posterior inferior cerebellar artery

C left anterior carotid artery

D right anterior carotid artery

E right middle carotid artery

## Question 9

A 47-year-old man presented to the Casualty department following sudden onset of left posterior auricular pain while in his garage working under his car. On examination he had a degree of neck pain and stiffness and also impaired coordination of the left hand and weakness and increased tone in his right limbs.

What is the most likely diagnosis?

A cervical dislocation

B migraine

C subarachnoid haemorrhage

D tension headache

E vertebral artery dissection

## Question 10

A 40-year-old woman is referred to you complaining of a three month history of dizziness, a 'buzzing noise' in her left ear and pain over her left cheek. The dizziness is intermittent in nature and usually lasts for up to two minutes. She describes the pain in her cheek as occurring intermittently several times a day, like an electric shock, and lasting several seconds each time. Over the last two weeks, she has also noticed mild difficulty closing her left eyelid and her friends have commented that her face is slightly asymmetrical. On examination, she looks relatively anxious. Cranial nerve examination reveals a reduced left corneal reflex, mild difficulty in closing the eyelids of her left eye and a slight droop over the left side of her face when she is asked to smile. Hallpike's manoeuvre is negative. Weber's test reveals lateralisation of the sound to the right ear. Rinne's test reveals air conduction better than bone conduction in both ears. The rest of the neurological examination is unremarkable.

What is the most likely diagnosis?

A acoustic neuroma

B craniopharyngioma

C glomus jugulare tumour

D parasagittal meningioma

E prolactinoma

## Question 11

A 60-year-old woman presented with three months' history of diplopia and blurred vision of left eye. She denied any pain or other neurological symptoms. Her previous medical history was unremarkable. Her pulse was 84 regular, and blood pressure 120/72. She smoked 20 cigarettes per day and apparently drank alcohol in moderation. Her general medical examination was normal. Her visual acuity on the right was 6/6 and on the left 6/36. There was a left partial ptosis and a mild proptosis with conjunctival injection. The left pupil was smaller than the right but was reacting normally to light. There was some limitation of abduction of the left eye. Fundoscopy showed a pale left optic disk. The left corneal reflex was reduced. The remainder of the neurological examination was normal. Routine blood tests including full blood count, serum urea and electrolytes, liver function tests, thyroid function, serum calcium, serum creatine kinase, and autoantibody screen were normal. Her electrocardiogram and chest radiograph showed no abnormalities. Slit lamp examination was normal and intra-ocular pressures were within normal range.

Where is the most likely anatomical focus of her symptoms?

A cavernous sinus

B superior orbital fissure

C orbital apex syndrome

D optic chiasm

E brainstem

## Question 12

A 42-year-old woman is admitted with a headache, mild photophobia and low grade fever. Two months previously, she had been on a walking holiday in southern Germany. Two days following admission, she develops a right lower motor neurone facial palsy. The CSF has 175 cells per $mm^3$ (over 90% lymphocytes), protein 1.2 g/L and a glucose that is just less than two-thirds serum glucose; oligoclonal bands are present.

The most likely diagnosis is:

A Behcet's disease

B HIV infection

C Lyme disease

D multiple sclerosis

E neurosarcoidosis

## Question 13

A 17-year-old girl presented with a two day history of severe back pain. A plain x-ray film of her spine was normal. Two days later, she complained of tingling in her fingers and toes. The next day she became generally weak. She presented in Accident and Emergency, where on examination, she had bilateral lower motor neurone facial weakness, tetraparesis with weakness in all limbs (4/5), areflexia, flexor plantars and normal sensation. A lumbar puncture was performed and the cerebrospinal fluid (CSF) analysis showed:

| | |
|---|---|
| CSF protein | 1.4 g/L |
| CSF glucose | normal |
| CSF cell count | 0 |

What is the most likely diagnosis?

A botulism

B Guillain-Barré syndrome

C acute poliomyelitis

D myasthenia gravis

E conversion disorder

## Question 14

A previously well 46-year-old successful trader presents with a two day history of progressively worsening headaches, dizziness, double vision, dry mouth and swallowing difficulties. His wife has also noticed that his face has been slightly asymmetrical over the last day or so. He denies any sensory or gastrointestinal symptoms. Three days ago, he injured his left hand while gardening and the wound on his little finger is red and tender. He admitted also, in confidence, that he did enjoy occasionally using recreational drugs. On examination, he is alert and orientated. Observations are: the pulse is 60 beats/min, blood pressure 130/65 mmHg, temperature 38°C. He has ptosis, large poorly reactive pupils, diplopia on looking to the extremities horizontally bilaterally, weakness of closing the eyelids (right worse than left) and inability to whistle properly. He also chokes when asked to swallow a little water. Power is mildly generally reduced in the upper limbs and lower limbs. Deep tendon reflexes are generally depressed and sensation is normal.

**Investigations reveal:**

| | |
|---|---|
| haemoglobin | 14.0 g/L |
| white cell count | $10 \times 10^9$/L |
| platelet count | $200 \times 10^9$/L |
| serum sodium | 139 mmol/L |
| serum potassium | 4.0 mmol/L |
| serum urea | 6.8 mmol/L |
| plasma glucose | 7.5 mmol/L |

**Cerebrospinal fluid:**

| | |
|---|---|
| CSF opening pressure | 15 cm |
| CSF cell count | < 2 per mm$^3$ |
| CSF protein | 0.3 g/L |
| CSF glucose | 6.1 mmol/L |

What is the most likely diagnosis?

A botulism

B Guillain-Barré syndrome

C Lyme disease

D myaesthenia gravis

E tetanus

## Question 15

An 18-year-old female presented with bilateral ptosis and tiredness towards afternoons. She had a short tensilon (edrophonium) test which was positive. A diagnosis of myasthenia gravis was made and she was started on pyridostigmine. She now subsequently relapses and is given edrophonium intravenously. However, her condition deteriorates and her forced expiratory volume falls to 1.0. She is transferred to the High Dependency Unit. An initial CT scan and chest x-ray are normal.

What should be the next management step?

A azathioprine

B emergency thymectomy

C intravenous methylprednisolone

D neostigmine

E plasma exchange

## Question 16

A 45-year-old woman presented with a six month history of slurring of her speech, expressionless face, right partial ptosis and diplopia. All her symptoms are worse in the evening.

What is the most appropriate diagnostic clinical examination?

A count numbers from one to fifty aloud

B demonstration of diminished reflexes

C demonstration of tongue fasciculations

D gait

E pupillary reaction to light

## Question 17

A 60-year-old man presents with an episode of memory loss. His mood, according to his wife, had always been 'excellent'. Three days previously, he had become markedly confused. His wife led him into the house – he apparently sat down at her request, and had a cup of tea. He then wandered around the house, carrying his cup of tea around and remaining confused, and able to have some conversation with his wife, though continuing to ask similar questions repeatedly. Speech and gait were noted to be normal by the wife. After three hours, he abruptly returned to normal, and had absolutely no recollection of the events. Previous medical history was unremarkable, and he had previously retired from management due to problems at work, having sustained this job since 18. Smoking and drinking histories were unremarkable, apart from a couple of whiskies per night as a 'night-cap'. There had been no history of trauma. His wife was most concerned that her husband was suffering from a prodromal form of Alzheimer's disease. There was a 'soft' family history of Alzheimer's disease in his family.

The most likely diagnosis is:

**A** alcoholic related amnesia

**B** chronic subdural haematoma

**C** prodromal form of Alzheimer's disease

**D** hysterical fugue state

**E** transient global amnesia

## Question 18

A 70-year-old man is referred with a six month history of increasing unsteadiness. He describes an irregular swaying gait with a tendency to drift to the right when walking. His wife comments that he tends to keep his feet apart when standing. In addition he has noticed problems with urinary urgency and frequency. Multiple urine samples sent by his GP have failed to detect infection. His muscles sometimes feel stiff but he puts this down to old age. On examination, pulse is 72 beats/min, BP 140/85 mmHg lying, 110/60 mmHg standing. Higher cognitive testing was unremarkable. The muscles of the upper and lower limbs show increased tone in the opposing muscle groups when the joints are passively moved. There is no obvious loss of muscle bulk. Power appears to be normal in all muscle groups. Gait is broad-based, with a tendency to lean to the right. Reflexes are brisk throughout and plantar responses are downgoing bilaterally. Finger-to-nose testing is impaired in the upper limbs. Sensory examination is unremarkable.

What is the most likely diagnosis?

A amyotrophic lateral sclerosis

B chronic inflammatory demyelinating polyneuropathy

C Friedreich's ataxia

D multiple system atrophy

E normal pressure hydrocephalus

## Question 19

A 60-year-old man presented with a 2-year history of forgetfulness, attentional difficulties, and paroxysmal drowsiness. He was examined by the GP who recorded bilateral bradykinesia and rigidity in the upper limbs. He was subsequently started on L-dopa. Six weeks later he developed visual hallucinations. The visual hallucinations persisted, despite stopping the L-dopa. The GP had started him on a small dose of haloperidol (5 mg). However, the patient developed severe vomiting and drowsiness; he recovered when haloperidol was discontinued. He had little facial expression, mild bradykinesia and rigidity in the upper limbs with a resting tremor of the left arm. Gait was normal. His MMSE was 20/30. The remainder of the neurological examination was normal.

**Investigations revealed:**

**Blood tests:**

| | |
|---|---|
| haemoglobin | 16.5 g/L |
| white cell count | $8.9 \times 10^9$/L |
| platelet count | $294 \times 10^9$/L |
| serum sodium | 139 mmol/L |
| serum potassium | 4.3 mmol/L |
| serum urea | 6.7 mmol/L |
| serum creatinine | 91 µmol/L |
| serum albumin | 39 g/L |
| serum total bilirubin | 19 µmol/L |
| serum aspartate aminotransferase | 28 U/L |
| serum alkaline phosphatase | 99 U/L |
| serum calcium (corrected) | 2.4 mmol/L |
| plasma glucose | 4.2 mmol |
| free T4 | 11 pmol |
| free T3 | 8 pmol |
| plasma thyroid-stimulating hormone | 3 mU |
| serum vitamin $B_{12}$ | 228 ng |
| **VDRL:** | negative |

**Further tests:**

| | |
|---|---|
| **CT head:** | normal |
| **EEG:** | normal |

What is the most likely diagnosis?

A idiopathic Parkinson's disease

B diffuse Lewy body disease

C Alzheimer's disease

D schizophrenia

E vascular dementia

## Question 20

A 35-year-old man is referred because of increasing concerns about his mood and change of personality. He has become depressed and apathetic. He is irritable and is noted to have poor memory and concentration. Examination reveals that he is extremely fidgety, has poor balance and tends to avert gaze. Saccadic eye movements are made with simultaneous head thrusts. There is no limb or facial dystonia.

The most likely diagnosis is:

A schizophrenia

B neuroleptic-induced dyskinesia

C Wilson's disease (hepatolenticular degeneration)

D systemic lupus erythematosus

E Huntington's disease

## Question 21

A 25-year-old is referred because of a progressively worsening ataxia. Ten months previously he had been noted to have become withdrawn and low in mood. Six months ago he complained of painful sensations in the limbs, but clinical examination was normal. On examination now, there are frequent widespread involuntary movements that are considered to be myoclonic jerks, made worse by sudden sounds. He has profound limb ataxia and mild dysarthria.

The most likely diagnosis is:

A progressive spinocerebellar ataxia (SCA) syndrome

B new variant Creutzfeld-Jacob disease (CJD)

C sporadic CJD

D multiple system atrophy

E paraneoplastic cerebellar degeneration

## Question 22

A 78-year-old man presented with an unsteady (wide-based) gait. He was noted to be becoming impaired with his memory and agitated at nights. His GP started him on an antidepressant, and wished to rule out a diagnosis of dementia. He was incontinent of urine. He was a heavy smoker and had lost 2 stone in weight over the previous two months. His blood sugar was 10 mmol/L.

Which is the next best investigation?

A CT head

B chest film

C HbA1c

D thyroid function tests

E urinary spot sodium

## Question 23

A 60-year-old man has the clinical diagnosis of idiopathic Parkinson's disease. He is commenced on treatment with L-dopa and dopa decarboxylase inhibitor therapy. However, he continues to have a troublesome tremor.

Which of the following drugs would be most likely to help?

A amantadine

B trihexyphenyl (benzhexol)

C propanolol

D ropinirole

E selegiline

## Question 24

A 70-year-old male presents with irritation of legs, particularly at night, of six months' duration. He is aware of a vague irritation in both legs that keeps him awake for most of the night. He finds that rubbing his legs or walking around gives him some relief but the problem has deteriorated over the last two months, and he is getting little sleep due to this problem. He has a past history of hypertension, for which he takes atenolol and ramipril, and he is on no other medication. He stopped smoking 10 years ago and drinks little alcohol. On examination, he has a blood pressure of 148/88 mmHg. No abnormalities are found on neurological examination of the legs. Both plantars are flexor, muscle power is normal and sensation is intact.

Which of the following is the most appropriate management for this patient?

A start amitryptiline

B start bromocriptine

C start phenytoin

D stop atenolol

E stop ramipril

## Question 25

A 62-year-old man presented with difficulty in walking. He had been admitted to hospital where he was diagnosed as 'off legs', and treated for a urinary tract infection. He had a past history of diabetes mellitus and cervical spondylosis, which had required surgical decompression eight years previously. He drank 20 units of alcohol weekly. On examination, there was fasciculation, wasting and weakness in the left deltoid and biceps, with weakness in the shoulder girdle muscles bilaterally. There was fasciculation in the glutei and quadriceps bilaterally, weakness of hip flexion and foot dorsiflexion, brisk reflexes in the upper and lower limbs, and extensor plantar responses. There was no sensory impairment.

The most likely diagnosis is:

A alcoholic myopathy

B thoracic meningioma

C motor neurone disease

D recurrent cervical cord compression

E syringomyelia

## Question 26

A 35-year-old woman presents complaining that she has repeatedly burnt her fingers inadvertently and is now developing numbness over her shoulders and arms. Examination demonstrates normal cranial nerves, diminished pin-prick sensation over the neck and arms down to the fingers with loss of deep tendon reflexes in the upper limbs. Proprioception is intact. In the legs, there is mild bilateral spasticity, power is full and sensation intact; deep tendon reflexes are brisk, and plantar responses extensor. The most likely diagnosis is:

A alcoholic myopathy

B thoracic meningioma

C motor neurone disease

D recurrent cervical cord compression

E syringomyelia

## Question 27

A 17-year-old woman presented with ataxia, dysarthria and incoordination of her upper limbs since the age of 10. She is now wheelchair bound. On examination, she has scanning speech, gaze-evoked horizontal nystagmus, ataxia of upper limbs, spastic paraparesis with absent knee and ankle reflexes, extensor plantar response, and bilateral pes cavus. What is the diagnosis?

A ataxia telangiectasia

B autosomal dominant spinocerebellar ataxia

C brainstem glioma

D Friedreich's ataxia

E multiple sclerosis

## Question 28

A 26-year-old woman with ptosis, weakness, a pacemaker *in situ* and cataracts, gave birth to a boy who had hypotonia and required resuscitation and subsequently assisted ventilation. The likely diagnosis of the mother is:

A syphilis

B dystrophia myotonica

C galactosaemia

D Hurler's syndrome

E hypothyroidism

## Question 29

A 36-year-old woman went to the South of France to visit the museum at Monte Carlo. She woke up with severe pain around the right shoulder one morning. A few days later she developed weakness of the right arm. At the same time the pain started to improve. She denied any injuries. Two weeks before her holiday she had suffered from an upper respiratory tract infection. On examination, she had weakness of right shoulder abduction, elbow flexion and reduced sensation over C5 and C6 dermatomes. The right biceps reflex was absent. Her previous medical history only included a lumpectomy for a breast malignancy, which was thought to have been successfully cleared. Her symptoms resolved after 2½ months.

What was the most likely diagnosis?

A C5 radiculopathy

B C6 radiculopathy

C axillary nerve palsy

D metastatic infiltration of the brachial plexus

E neuralgic amyotrophy

## Question 30

A 56-year-old female lawyer with long-standing rheumatoid arthritis presented with pain in the neck and radiating to the left hand, interfering with her work in Chambers. She herself noted wasting in the right hand muscles. She was well controlled on penicillamine. On examination there was inversion of the biceps and supinator reflex jerks. The triceps jerk was brisk. Knee reflexes were present. The plantars were equivocal because of rheumatoid arthritis of the hallux. Fasciculations were noted, neck movements were restricted, and position sense was slightly impaired at the elbow.

What is the most likely diagnosis?

A atlanto-axial subluxation

B vitamin $B_{12}$ deficiency

C cervical cord tumour

D cervical myelopathy

E motor neurone disease

## Question 31

A 35-year-old man presented with shooting pain of the lateral aspect of his left arm. On examination he had weakness of biceps with a diminished biceps reflex.

What is the most likely explanation of his symptoms?

A C5 radiculopathy

B C6 radiculopathy

C C7 radiculopathy

D C8 radiculopathy

E T1 radiculopathy

## Question 32

A 33-year-old male presents with marked haemetemesis. He is noted to have a pulse of 128/min and a blood pressure of 100/60 mmHg. He is immediately given a transfusion of three units of blood, an urgent endoscopy reveals a large duodenal ulcer which does not respond to injection therapy and he undergoes laparoscopy with oversew of his duodenal ulcer. He makes a good immediate post-operative recovery and receives treatment with omeprazole. No further bleeding is noted and his full blood count remains stable. However, on the twelfth post-operative day he notes persisting weakness of the right hand. On examination, there is wasting of the small muscles of the right hand.

What is the likely site of the lesion?

A wrist

B elbow

C neck

D brachial plexus

E cortex

## Question 33

A 46-year-old woman has had nocturnal pain and paraesthesiae in the right forearm and hand for six months. The symptoms typically wake her and she shakes the hand to relieve them. For several years, she had complained of neck pain, exacerbated by movement. She had smoked around 10 cigarettes a week for the previous two years. Examination demonstrated subtle thenar wasting, and very mild weakness of right abductor pollicis brevis.

What is the most likely diagnosis?

A C6 radiculopathy

B carpal tunnel syndrome

C Pancoast's (lung apex) syndrome

D thoracic outlet (cervical rib) syndrome

E ulnar nerve compression at the elbow

## Question 34

A 50-year-old man presented with tingling in the left upper limb, which he noticed predominantly at night time. The pain was reported to have originated in the neck and radiated down the left arm. He proceeded to have numbness and paraesthesiae in the left lower limb. On examination he had restriction of neck movements and there was mild wasting noted in the left biceps. There was inversion of the supinator and biceps jerks. His knee jerks and ankle jerks were exaggerated bilaterally and he had a positive extensor plantar response. He then developed paraesthesia and numbness of the right lower limb. A diagnosis of cord compression was made and he underwent a surgical decompression. The post-operative period was complicated by septicaemia and urinary tract infection and he remained in bed for four days. He subsequently developed inability to dorsiflex his right foot and right big toe. There was numbness on the outside of the foot and there was decreased eversion, but inversion was normal. His reflexes remained as before.

What is the cause of the problem?

A common peroneal nerve palsy

B L4 root lesion

C recurrence of the original cord compression

D sacral plexopathy

E sciatic nerve palsy

## Question 35

A 60-year-old man presented with acute weakness and pain of his right lower limb. He had awoken one morning after playing football with his grandson and had been aware of marked pain and weakness of his right leg. On examination there was weakness of ankle dorsiflexion, plantar flexion, eversion and inversion, and thigh abduction and extension.

What is the most likely diagnosis?

A common peroneal nerve palsy

B L4 root lesion

C recurrence of the original cord compression

D sacral plexopathy

E sciatic nerve palsy

## Question 36

A 30-year-old man who had been under much stress at work because of an impending take-over bid presented with a one-week history of severe constant pain behind the right eye, which he described like a 'huge drill' radiating across his right frontotemporal region, waking him at 2 a.m. every morning, lasting 90 minutes. He also noted that his right eye is watery and red during the attacks, along with the feeling of a blocked right nostril. On examination during an attack, there was a partial right sided ptosis with meiosis of the pupil. The blood pressure was 130/70, and his GCS was 15/15.

What is the most appropriate treatment during the attacks?

A amitryptiline

B indomethacin

C pethidine

D tramadol

E sumatriptan

## Question 37

A 22-year-old obese woman presented with an eight week history of headaches, pulsatile tinnitus and transient visual loss on standing lasting a few seconds. She had otherwise been well, with no history of note. She took the oral contraceptive pill and had been taking this for the last six months, also using salbutamol inhalers on an occasional basis for the asthma which she had from childhood. She also took vitamin A supplements which she bought over the counter for her general health. On examination, the only abnormality of note was bilateral papilloedema. MRI brain and MRV (MR venogram) were normal. Lumbar puncture showed an opening pressure of 38, normal protein, glucose, and cells.

What is the most likely diagnosis?

A herpes simplex encephalitis

B intracranial hypertension secondary to vitamin A

C malignant meningitis

D sagittal sinus thrombosis secondary to OCP

E frontal meningioma

## Question 38

A 34-year-old female presents to her GP with a left-sided excruciating throbbing headache. She reports having to hold her head, and she has periods of soreness in between attacks. She normally has attacks lasting 40 minutes, and finds her eyelid drooping over a swollen left eye. Her GP has prescribed indomethacin, which completely stops the headache. She has kept a diary of her attacks, and this diary reveals a mean number of headaches of around 20. According to her partner, she has been becoming increasingly anxious about the fact that the headaches may be a symptom of something 'sinister'.

The most likely diagnosis is:

A cluster headache

B trigeminal neuralgia

C episodic paroxysmal hemicrania

D tension headache

E migraine

## Question 39

A 20-year-old woman has a history of paroxysmal episodes of dysarthria, ataxia and diplopia lasting for 20–30 minutes followed by right-sided severe headache associated with vomiting, lasting for 1–3 days. The episodes occur once every month. MRI brain and MRA (angiogram) are normal.

What is the most likely diagnosis?

A basilar artery TIAs

B basilar migraine

C brainstem arteriovenous malformation

D giant cell arteritis

E multiple sclerosis

## Question 40

A 55-year-old man with poorly controlled hypertension presented with headache and right-sided weakness. He was right-handed. The CT scan revealed a left-sided intracerebral haematoma in the frontoparietal area. The blood pressure measured 160/90 mmHg. The Glasgow Coma Scale was 15/15. The patient's condition had remained unchanged for two hours.

What is the appropriate management?

A control of blood pressure immediately

B neurosurgical referral

C intravenous mannitol

D observe

E dexamethasone

## Question 41

A 60-year-old woman, a smoker of 30 years history (around 10 cigarettes a day), presented with an acute severe occipital headache, unsteadiness in her gait and vomiting. She had a history of poorly controlled hypertension. On examination, there was nystagmus to the left, and ataxia of the left limbs and gait.

The most likely diagnosis is:

A acute cerebellar haemorrhage

B basal ganglia haemorrhage

C pontine haemorrhage

D subdural haemorrhage

E temporal lobe haemorrhage

## Question 42

A 38-year-old man presents with an episode of right-sided weakness affecting his right arm and leg. The weakness occurred while he was eating breakfast and resolved completely in 30 minutes. Three months earlier he had an episode of slurred speech lasting a few minutes and had been investigated extensively in hospital. Aspirin 75 mg had been started as treatment. On examination, he is overweight with a BMI of 38, pulse 88/min regular and BP 140/85 mmHg. Heart sounds are normal and no carotid bruits are detectable. The neurological examination is unremarkable except for an upgoing plantar response on the right side. A Doppler ultrasound of the carotid arteries reveals 50% stenosis in the proximal carotid arteries bilaterally.

What evidence-based intervention is most likely to prevent further episodes of the patient's condition?

A add clopidogrel to aspirin

B add dipyridamole to aspirin

C increase the dose of aspirin to 150 mg daily

D stop aspirin, and start clopidogrel alone

E stop aspirin, and start dipyridamole alone

## Question 43

A 21-year-old woman presented with a six week history of fever, headaches and general malaise. One week prior to admission, she had an episode of loss of consciousness, which was accompanied by urinary incontinence and transient weakness of the left hand. On examination, she was drowsy and there was rigidity of neck movements. She had a temperature of 38.4°C. The blood pressure was 120/80 mmHg. There were no focal neurological signs. On inspection of the oral cavity, there were white plaques over the tonsils and pharynx. Examination of the heart, lungs and abdomen was normal.

**Investigations revealed:**

| | |
|---|---|
| **CT brain:** | normal |
| **Cerebrospinal fluid:** | |
| opening pressure | 23 cm $H_2O$ |
| cells | 120/$mm^3$ (all lymphocytes) |
| protein | 1.4 g/L |
| glucose | 1.4 mmol/L (blood glucose = 5.1 mmol/L) |
| gram stain | negative |
| ZN stain | negative |

Which of the following investigations will best confirm the likely diagnosis?

A CSF protein immunoelectrophoresis

B Indian ink stain on CSF

C CSF ELISA for TB antigen

D CSF pyruvate estimation

E blood cultures

## Question 44

A 55-year-old man presented with 6-month history of fatiguable proximal weakness of both upper and lower limbs, dry mouth and impotence. He was a heavy smoker of 30 cigarettes per day and drank 12 units of alcohol per week. Otherwise he had been well. On examination, he demonstrated digital clubbing, was an obese individual with a blood pressure of 155/90 mmHg and was apyrexial. Chest heart and abdominal examination were normal. There was proximal weakness grade 4/5 in both upper and lower limbs. The reflexes were generally depressed. Plantars were flexor and sensation was normal. He had also complained of blurred vision and a dry mouth. A full blood count was normal, and anti-ACh receptor antibody was negative. What is the most likely diagnosis?

A Lambert-Eaton myaesthenic syndrome

B motor neurone disease

C peripheral motor neuropathy

D myasthenia gravis

E polymyositis

## Question 45

A 39-year-old male dentist presents to the neurology clinic with twitching muscles. He has been particularly concerned about involuntary twitches that he has noticed in his muscles over the last six months. He is aware of these twitches particularly at night and when at rest. He plays tennis three times per week and notices that the twitches are worse after exercise. He has noticed no deterioration in his ability to exercise and his fitness has improved over the last three months. He is otherwise fit and well and takes no medication. His weight has been stable. He drinks approximately two bottles of wine per week but does not smoke.

On examination, he appears fit and well with a blood pressure of 122/78 mmHg. Cardiovascular, respiratory and abdominal examination are all normal. Neurological examination reveals normal tone and bulk but sporadic fasciculations are seen in the quadriceps, brachioradialis, biceps, triceps, calves and pectoralis muscles. No fasciculations are seen in the tongue. He is generally strong in all muscle groups tested, with 5/5 strength. Reflexes are all preserved with flexor plantar responses. Sensation is intact. Investigations are normal. What is the likely diagnosis?

A alcohol-related myopathy

B amyotrophic lateral sclerosis

C benign fasciculation syndrome

D chronic poliomyelitis

E hypokalaemic periodic paralysis

## Question 46

A 24-year-old woman presented with horizontal diplopia over the last six weeks. Three years ago she had a painful visual loss of the left eye, which recovered completely over the next three months. On examination, on looking to the right, there is loss of adduction of the left eye and nystagmus of the abducting eye. She has also noticed that her legs have become weaker, yet stiffer. On one occasion, she took a bath, and noted an unpleasant electric shock sensation which radiated down her back into her legs.

What is the underlying diagnosis?

A brainstem glioma

B brainstem stroke

C Friedreich's ataxia

D multiple sclerosis

E Wernicke's encephalopathy

## Question 47

A 30-year-old man presented with painless visual loss of his left eye over 24 hours. In two weeks he lost the vision of his right eye. There was no improvement of his visual acuity over the next two months. He denied any other symptoms. His previous medical history was unremarkable. He smokes 10 cigarettes per day and drinks around 20 units of alcohol per week. There is no relevant family history. He does not take any drugs. General medical examination is normal. His visual acuity is 6/60 on the right and finger counting on the left. His colour vision is impaired in both eyes. He has bilateral optic atrophy. The remainder of his neurological examination is normal. Blood tests including full blood count, serum urea and electrolytes, liver and thyroid function tests, bone function tests, serum glucose, autoantibody screen, VDRL, vitamin $B_{12}$ and folate are normal. CXR is normal. MRI brain and orbits are normal. CSF analysis is unremarkable.

What is the most likely diagnosis?

A multiple sclerosis

B alcohol/tobacco toxic induced optic neuropathy

C Leber's optic atrophy

D giant cell arteritis/ischaemic optic neuropathy

E glaucoma

## Question 48

A 72-year-old woman with a 2 week history of general malaise and weight loss presents with a painless, sudden-onset deterioration of vision in the right eye. Examination reveals a right afferent papillary defect, visual acuity of 6/36 in the right eye and a pale swollen optic disc. The erythrocyte sedimentation rate is 55 mm/hour (Westergren).

Which of the following management plans in your opinion is most appropriate?

A she requires an urgent carotid Doppler ultrasound

B a fluorescein angiogram should be immediately performed

C intravenous heparin should be commenced

D she should be started on high dose corticosteroids

E urgent MRI of the orbits should be required

## Question 49

A 55-year-old woman presents with headache, photophobia, nausea and vomiting, as well as blurred vision in her left eye. On examination, the eye is red, the pupil is oval and fixed (not responding to light or accommodation), and the cornea appears cloudy. Visual acuity is limited to finger counting.

Whilst waiting for an ophthalmology referral, which of the following would be a reasonable option?

A administer intravenous mannitol

B apply local pressure to the eyeball

C administer pilocarpine drops to the eye

D give oral beta blockers

E give intravenous atropine

## Question 50

A 44-year-old HIV seropositive patient is seen in a routine outpatient appointment. He was diagnosed with HIV disease two years ago when he presented with *Pneumocystis carinii* pneumonia (PCP) with a CD4 T-lymphocyte count of 40 cells/mm$^3$. After being treated for PCP he was started on combination antiretroviral therapy. His initial response to antiretroviral therapy had been promising, with an increase in his CD4 count (210 cells/mm$^3$) and achieving an undetectable HIV viral load in the peripheral blood.

One year ago, his CD4 count started to fall and HIV RNA became detectable in peripheral blood. An HIV viral resistance test confirmed resistance to all of his antiretroviral drugs. The patient admitted that over the preceeding three months he had only been taking his therapy intermittently. Despite the risks, he decided that he did not wish to have any further antiretroviral therapy. At this point, his CD4 count was 20 cells/mm$^3$ with a very high HIV viral load of 120 000 copies/mL. Seven months ago he presented with malaise, weight loss (8 kg), fevers and night sweats. *Mycobacterium avium intracellulare* (MAI) was isolated from a blood culture and he was started on therapy with ethambutol and rifabutin. He subsequently agreed to re-start antiretroviral therapy.

During his clinic consultation, he states that he has noticed a steady deterioration in his visual acuity over the past four weeks. His current medications include stavudine (d4T), didanosine (ddI), nevirapine, ethambutol, and rifabutin.

On examination, fundoscopy is normal. His last CD4 count, taken one month ago was 30 cells/mm$^3$, with an HIV viral load of 2500 copies/mL.

What is the most likely cause of his reduction in visual acuity?

A antiretroviral therapy

B cytomegalovirus retinitis

C ethambutol

D HIV retinopathy

E toxoplasma retinitis

## Question 51

A 28-year-old man presents to the acute medical on-call with an atypical pneumonia. However, his previous medical notes state that he has had a history of compulsive hand washing, with voices telling him to do so. He has been feeling depressed recently, in that he has become totally anhedonic concerning his job, about which his boss had said he was extremely apathetic. He appears unkempt, coherent, but with blunted affect. He admits to having consumed five pints of strong beer within the last 10 hours, and to cannabis use over the previous three years.

The most likely diagnosis is:

A substance misuse

B obsessive-compulsive disorder

C bipolar affective disorder

D schizophrenia

E schizoaffective disorder

## Question 52

A 31-year-old woman is referred to Outpatients by her GP for investigation of pain in the small joints of the hands. Apart from Raynaud's phenomenon, she is otherwise well.

Clinical examination is unremarkable. Routine full blood count, serum urea and electrolyes, LFTs, erythrocyte sedimentation rate are all normal. She is negative for rheumatoid factor, but ANA +ve 1/100 homogenous.

She is given a 6 month follow-up appointment and advised to take ibuprofen on an as-needed (PRN) basis. Twelve weeks later she presents to the Accident and Emergency Department with diplopia and blurred vision. She had been vomiting for the previous three weeks, and lost three kilograms in weight. She also complains of parasthesiae affecting the right hand and forearm.

On examination, her pulse is 90 regular, BP 105/73 mmHg. She is kept under observation for 48 hours, does not improve, and is referred back to rheumatology. She is then on examination apyrexial, has nystagmus in all directions with limited horizontal and vertical eye movements. Apart from finger/nose and heel/shin ataxia, neurological examination is normal. The Casualty consultant had performed the following tests:

| | |
|---|---|
| serum sodium | 134 mmol/L |
| serum potassium | 4 mmol/L |
| serum urea | 3 mmol/L |
| serum creatinine | 64 µmol/L |
| serum alkaline phosphatase | 234 U/L |
| serum aspartate transaminase | 231 U/L |
| serum albumin | 32 g/L |
| haemoglobin | 10.3 g/L, normochromic normocytic |
| platelet count | $345 \times 10^9$/L |
| complement components C3, C4 | 115% normal |
| anti-nuclear factor | positive |
| erythrocyte sedimentation rate | 44 mm/hr (Westergren) |
| serum C-reactive protein | 5 mg/L |

The most likely underlying diagnosis for the neurological symptoms is:

A systemic lupus erythematosus

B hypothyroidism

C Wernicke's encephalopathy

D pregnancy

E none of the above

## Question 53

A 40-year-old man with chronic alcohol abuse presented in the Accident and Emergency Department with confusion, agitation and ataxia. He had been found wandering the streets at 2 a.m. and was brought in by the police. He had been admitted on numerous occasions previously, related to alcohol abuse. On examination he appeared dishevelled, confused and smelt of alcohol. He was disoriented in time and place, with a mini-mental score of 16/30. He was apyrexial with a blood pressure of 138/90 mmHg. He had bilateral sixth nerve palsies, gaze-evoked nystagmus and gait ataxia.

What treatment should this patient receive?

A diazepam

B immunoglobulins

C further alcohol

D steroids

E thiamine

## Question 54

A 19-year-old lady is admitted with difficulty in swallowing: 36 hours previously she had taken an overdose of metoclopramide. Over the previous three hours, she had developed progressively worse dysphagia and drooling. She also complained of blurred vision. On examination, she was distressed but alert. There was drooping of the left side of her mouth. Her left eye was deviated to the left. The rest of her cranial nerve examination was normal.

The treatment of choice in this patient is:

A adrenaline

B chlorpheniramine

C hydrocortisone

D prochlorperazine

E procyclidine

## Question 55

A 52-year-old man comes to the Outpatient clinic with his wife. Over the last two months, he complains of hearing strange noises and occasionally non-threatening voices. His wife says that he also hears 'music'. On more detailed questioning, he admits to becoming more withdrawn recently and having spent most of his time now 'doing nothing'. His sleep is poor and he commonly wakes up at 2–3 a.m. His appetite has fallen off and he is eating very little, consequently losing about 10 kg in the last three months. He admits to drinking one and a half bottles of whisky a day. During the conversation, he appears calm, his speech is clear and articulate, but his attention is poor. He has no tremor. His three-minute recall of a given address is impaired. He does not exhibit any clouding of consciousness and there is no suggestion of delusions or paranoid symptoms.

What is the most likely diagnosis in this man?

A alcoholic hallucinosis

B Korsakoff's psychosis

C major depression with psychosis

D psychotic depression

E schizophrenia

## Question 56

A 48-year-old man with a known history of schizophrenia is admitted following increasing stiffness in his arms and jaws. He has been on fluphenazine for approximately two years. On examination, his pulse is 90 beats/minute, blood pressure 175/80 mmHg, and temperature 38.8°C. Neurological examination reveals generalised increased tone.

**Investigations reveal:**

| | |
|---|---|
| haemoglobin | 13.4 g/L |
| white cell count | $5 \times 10^9$/L |
| platelet count | $210 \times 10^9$/L |
| erythrocyte sedimentation rate | 5 mm/hr (Westergren) |
| serum sodium | 146 mmol/L |
| serum potassium | 3.7 mmol/L |
| serum urea | 7.3 mmol/L |
| serum creatinine | 72 μmol/L |

What treatment will you consider for his condition?

A benztropine

B bromocriptine

C lithium

D prednisolone

E procyclidine

# Answers to Chapter 10: Neurology, ophthalmology and psychiatry

These solutions aim to provide the reason(s) for the right answer, and also the reason(s) for the wrong answers being excluded.

1 **Answer D:** The most likely option is D, because of the patient's age, history of personality and behaviour change, and high MMSE score. Supporting evidence is his new liking for sweet foods. The family history for Parkinson's disease is not strong enough here for this to be a realistic option, although there is a variant of frontotemporal dementia associated with Parkinson's disease. His mood is good, and he has made no response to anti-depressants, making the major differential diagnosis of depression unlikely. Furthermore, as he reports no memory deficits and his MMSE is high, Alzheimer's disease is unlikely. Old age would not give you the changes in personality and behaviour reported. For a brief description of typical cases of the frontal variant of frontotemporal dementia, *see* Rahman et al. *Brain* (1999).

2 **Answer C:** His $CO_2$ retention is likely to be due to CNS depression and reduction in diaphragmatic contraction secondary to baclofen toxicity. Onset of toxicity is rapid and its effect can last up to 35–40 hours post ingestion. Features include drowsiness, coma, respiratory depression, hyporeflexia, hypotonia, hypothermia and hypotension. Bradycardia with first degree heart block and prolongation of Q-T interval can occur. Treatment is usually supportive and often requires intensive care. The presence of hypoxic drive is unlikely, in view of the patient being a non-smoker; thus, a reduction in inspired oxygen would not increase his respiratory drive. NIPPV would be an option but not in a patient with a GCS 8/15. Patients with a high risk of aspiration pneumonia are a contraindication to non-invasive ventilation. Doxapram has no place in the treatment of baclofen toxicity, nor in the treatment of type II respiratory failure in general.

3 **Answer D:** The answer here, as revealed by the symptoms and the high CK, is hypothyroidism.

4 **Answer E:** The presence of severe flinging movements indicates hemiballistic movements. The site of lesion is the contralateral subthalamic nucleus. The commonest cause is stroke. Usually the flinging movements stop spontaneously within 4–8 weeks. Tetrabenazine is the treatment of choice.

5 **Answer A:** Women on anticonvulsant therapy are advised to plan their pregnancies carefully so that any adjustments in therapy can be made prior to becoming pregnant. Ideally, reducing switching therapy should be done over a period of several months. Anticonvulsant agents are likely to produce foetal

malformations before 13 weeks. Therefore, the best option at this stage is to continue her current therapy.

6 **Answer A:** This is a classical history of Holmes-Adie pupil, of a large pupil which reacts sluggishly to light. There is normally delayed constriction in response to near vision, and accommodation may also be impaired. There is sometimes segmental palsy and spontaneous movement of the iris. Absent ankle jerks is sometimes an associated finding.

7 **Answer D:** This patient has Horner's syndrome, consisting of miosis, ptosis, anhydrosis (and enophthalmos). Because the sympathetic plexus accompanying the internal carotid artery innervates sweat glands only to the medial forehead, facial anhydrosis does not occur significantly with post-ganglionic Horner's syndrome.

8 **Answer A:** The unifying diagnosis is Wallenberg's syndrome (otherwise known as the lateral medullary syndrome).

9 **Answer E:** The typical presentation of vertebral artery dissection is a young person (average age 40 years) with severe occipital headache and neck pain following a recent head or neck injury. The trauma is often trivial, but is usually associated with some form of cervical distortion. About 85% of patients develop focal neurological signs due to ischaemia of the brain stem or cerebellum. The commonest neurological manifestations are symptoms attributable to lateral medullary dysfunction (i.e. Wallenberg's syndrome). The vessel that is usually occluded is likely to be the posterior inferior cerebellar artery, a branch of the vertebral artery. (*See* **Learning point**.)

10 **Answer A:** The combination of sensorineural deafness, facial nerve palsy and cranial nerve V involvement suggests a cerebellopontine angle tumour, e.g. acoustic neuroma.

Craniopharyngiomas are more common in children than in adults. Patients usually present with signs of local compression, especially of the visual system, or hypothalamic dysfunction, for example diabetes insipidus or growth failure. Glomus jugulare tumours tend to present with pulsatile tinnitus and conductive deafness.

Cranial nerves IX, X and XI which run through the jugular foramen are also commonly affected to varying degrees. Cranial nerves VII and XII may be affected if the tumour enlarges sufficiently. Parasagittal meningiomas may produce seizures or be entirely asymptomatic, often growing to enormous size before they are discovered. Lesions that reach sufficient size may cause spastic paraparesis and incontinence. Prolactinomas commonly present with amenorrhoea and galactorrhoea in women and impotence in men. They are also associated with visual field defects.

11 **Answer C:** The combination of optic neuropathy, proptosis, chemosis, Horner's syndrome, ophthalmoplegia (in this case due to a sixth nerve palsy), and involvement of the first branch of the trigeminal nerve is typical of orbital apex syndrome. Proptosis and chemosis are useful signs to distinguish orbital apex syndrome from cavernous sinus pathology.

12 **Answer C:** Lyme disease is associated with various forms of cardiac (e.g. heart block) and neurological involvement, including Bell's palsy, mononeuritis multiplex, ataxia, myelitis, chorea or meningoencephalitis. Serum and CSF serological titres are often less reliable as a guide to diagnosis than demonstration of a typical tick bite wound.

13 **Answer B:** The clinical history is again very typical of Guillain-Barré syndrome. Back pain is very common and often severe enough to require opiate treatment. Acute onset of weakness with areflexia and high CSF protein with normal cell count are typical features of the condition.

14 **Answer A:** Botulism occurs either from gut colonisation (e.g. ingestion of contaminated home-canned food) or an infected wound. There is currently an epidemic of this condition in drug abusers. *Clostridium botulinum* spores are widespread in soil and aquatic sediment. The bacterium grows in anaerobic conditions (such as the necrotic injection sites of drug users). Typical initial features include diplopia, ptosis, facial weakness, dysarthria and dysphagia. Later, respiratory difficulty and limb weakness occur. Neuromuscular blockade causes the clinical features. In botulism, the impaired cholinergic transmission also involves autonomic synapses, causing poorly reactive dilated pupils, dry mouth, paralytic ileus and occasionally bradycardia. Reflexes are depressed or absent, sensation is normal and CSF is normal in botulism. In the Miller-Fisher variant of Guillain-Barré syndrome, CSF often shows elevated protein. Lyme disease tends to spare the extraocular muscles. Pupillary abnormalities do not occur in myasthenia gravis. In tetanus, clinical features include jaw stiffness, spasm of jaw muscles and hyperreflexia.

15 **Answer E:** The correct diagnosis is a myaesthenia crisis, i.e. an exacerbation of myaesthenia gravis. The treatment of choice is either intravenous immunoglobulins or plasma exchange. Transfer to ITU is essential because patients may deteriorate rapidly, requiring intubation and ventilation (around 10%). Those with artificial ventilation are not given cholinergics as this avoids stimulation of pulmonary secretions and uncertainties about overdosage.

16 **Answer A:** Another question on myasthenia gravis, a neurological autoimmune disease. It is characterised by fluctuating skeletal muscle weakness that worsens with use and improves with rest. Eye, facial, oropharyngeal, axial, and limb muscles may be involved in varying combinations and degree of severity.

The symptoms usually increase as the day progresses. The demonstration of fatigability is the cardinal feature of myasthenia gravis.

17 **Answer E:** This is typical of transient global amnesia (TGA), which represents a transient vascular insufficiency of both hippocampi, in general of the mesial temporal lobes, both of which have a common blood supply from the basilar artery or posterior cerebral artery trunk. Hypoglycaemic attacks, for example due to an insulinoma, are usually shorter lasting, and are associated with adrenergic features.

18 **Answer D:** Multiple system atrophy (a form of parkinsonian syndrome) is a neurodegenerative disorder characterised by parkinsonian features, autonomic insufficiency (leading to postural hypotension, anhydrosis, disturbance of sphincter control, impotence) and signs of a cerebellar deficit. Chronic inflammatory demyelinating polyneuropathy is clinically similar to Guillain-Barré syndrome (hyporeflexia or areflexia, paraesthesiae and mild sensory deficits in the upper and lower extremities, weakness) except that it follows a chronic progressive course. Friedreich's ataxia is characterised by progressive gait ataxia, depressed knee and ankle reflexes, cerebellar signs, and impairment of joint position and vibration sense – clinical manifestations almost always begin to appear before puberty. Normal pressure hydrocephalus is less likely because of the lack of cognitive impairment, although it is characterised also by unsteady gait and urinary problems.

19 **Answer B:** Diffuse Lewy body disease typically presents with dementia, parkinsonism, visual hallucinations, intermittent alteration of attention, and sensitivity to neuroleptics. Patients with idiopathic Parkinson's disease do not usually manifest visual hallucinations until many years after the introduction of L-dopa treatment (> 5 years). Dementia usually appears 5–10 years after the onset of parkinsonism.

20 **Answer E:** Personality changes often occur first in Huntington's disease, accompanied by other neuropsychiatric features such as depression. The simultaneous head thrusts with the saccadic eye movements, along with the finding that he is 'extremely fidgety' is suggestive of the diagnosis.

21 **Answer:** C: The duration and early onset of psychiatric symptoms make sporadic CJD the most likely diagnosis, and the presentation of myoclonic sounds (with an acoustic startle response) fits in with this.

22 **Answer A:** The triad of unsteady gait, memory impairment and urinary incontinence suggests the diagnosis of normal pressure hydrocephalus. CT head of the brain is the investigation of choice to show enlarged ventricles out of proportion to the overall extent of cerebral atrophy.

23 **Answer B:** Anticholinergic drugs such as benzhexol remain the treatment of choice in Parkinsonian tremor. L-dopa, selegiline and dopamine agonists are less effective in tremor.

24 **Answer B:** This patient has 'restless legs syndrome', a condition characterised by uncomfortable, irritating and sometimes painful sensations which usually occur in the legs when at rest and usually at night. The condition is benign and clinical examination usually reveals no abnormalities. It may be exacerbated by diuretics, tricyclic antidepressants, phenytoin and calcium antagonists. Studies suggest that dopamine agonists and L-Dopa may be useful treatments.

25 **Answer C:** There are mixed signs of lower (wasting, fasciculations) and upper (brisk reflexes, extensor plantar response) motor neurone involvement in the presence of normal sensation. Motor neurone disease is the commonest cause of such presentation. Alcoholic myopathy and diabetic myopathy do not share upper motor neurone signs. Syringomyelia presents with sensory symptoms and signs. One would expect sensory involvement with cervical cord compression.

26 **Answer E:** Syringomyelia usually progresses slowly; the course may extend over many years. It usually involves the cervical area. Symptomatic presentation depends primarily on the location of the lesion within the neuraxis. Clinical manifestations commonly include the following: (a) dissociated sensory loss (loss of pain and temperature sensation), while light touch, vibration, and position senses are preserved; (b) pain and temperature sensation may be impaired in either or both arms, or in 'cape-like' distribution across the shoulders and upper torso anteriorly and posteriorly; (c) diffuse muscle atrophy that begins in the hands and progresses proximally to include the forearms and shoulder girdles. This disease can also produce autonomic disturbances, and also a 'syringobulbia'.

Other manifestations include frequently painless ulcers of the hands, and also 'neurogenic arthropathies' (Charcot joints) which affect the shoulder, elbow, or wrist.

27 **Answer D:** Friedreich's ataxia is an autosomal recessive condition presenting in the first decade. It is associated with spinocerebellar degeneration. Bilateral pes cavus is common. The typical clinical signs are cerebellum dysfunction, spastic paraparesis, absent reflexes in lower limbs. Cardiomyopathy, diabetes and optic atrophy are also associated with this condition.

28 **Answer B:** All the clinical features given are of myotonic dystrophy (MD). This condition demonstrates the genetic phenomenon of anticipation, the tendency for a genetic disorder to become more severe and present at an earlier age in successive generations. Affected individuals with classical MD have

larger AGC or CTG mutations. Myotonic dystrophy is autosomal dominant, located on chromosome 19q13.3. The most severe form of MD is congenital MD, which presents at birth with intrauterine growth retardation, severe hypotonia, muscle weakness and feeding difficulties. Children with congenital MD have developmental delay, learning difficulties, and develop myotonia in their teens.

**29** **Answer E:** The clinical history is typical of neuralgic amyotrophy. It is usually preceded by an upper respiratory tract infection. Pain around the shoulder is the presenting symptom, often severe. Neuralgic amyotrophy is an inflammatory condition of the brachial plexus. Usually, as the pain starts resolving, weakness begins and affects the muscles innervated by the upper brachial plexus (C5–6). Treatment is conservative. It is usually a self-limiting condition (improvement over weeks to months). This cannot be an axillary nerve palsy as the findings are not restricted to the deltoid muscle. Neoplastic infiltration of the brachial plexus is also a consideration, but this would be progressive and produce on-going pain.

**30** **Answer D:** The presence of inversion of biceps and supinator reflexes indicating cervical myelopathy at C5, C6. This is a very important sign, which distinguishes cervical myelopathy from motor neurone disease.

**31** **Answer A:** Shooting pain is the cardinal symptom of a radiculopathy. The lateral aspect of the arm represents C5 dermatome. C5 innervates biceps, C6 brachioradialis, C7 triceps, C8 finger flexors, and T1 small muscles of the hand.

**32** **Answer B:** This is an entrapment ulnar neuropathy at the elbow (the commonest site for entrapment of ulnar nerve). A common complication in ill patients in hospital. Nerve conduction studies will confirm the site of the lesion.

**33** **Answer B:** The usual features of carpal tunnel syndrome are thenar wasting, weakness of opposition, abduction, and flexion of the thumb, and weakness of the index finger and middle lumbricals. Sensation is usually impaired over the palmar aspect of the lateral side of the hand, thumb, index finger, middle finger, and lateral radial border of the ring finger. The palm is spared as the palmar branch of the nerve lies superior to the retinaculum.

**34** **Answer A:** The commonest cause of acute foot drop after prolonged bed rest is entrapment common peroneal neuropathy at the neck of fibula. Typically there is weakness of ankle dorsiflexion, eversion, diminished sensation of the lateral aspect of leg and dorsum of foot. The ankle reflex remains intact.

**35 Answer D:** The most likely diagnosis is sacral plexopathy. Thigh abduction and extension weakness indicate gluteal medius and maximus involvement (L5, S1). This finding distinguishes it from the sciatic nerve palsy.

**36 Answer E:** The correct diagnosis is cluster headache ('migrainous neuralgia'). It is associated with lacrimation of the eye, ptosis, eyelid swelling, injection of the conjunctiva and nasal congestion. It usually presents in male patients (M/F 9:1), can occur at any age, and occurs in the early hours of the morning. The treatment of choice during acute attacks includes s/c sumatriptan; high flow oxygen (100%; 68 L/min) often produces relief within 10 minutes. Prophylactic treatment includes lithium, verapamil, sodium valproate, prednisolone and ergotamines.

**37 Answer B:** The findings are consistent with benign intracranial hypertension (papilloedema, normal CSF analysis, normal brain imaging). Vitamin A is a well known cause of this condition (as well as tetracycline and the oral contraceptive). (*See* **Learning point.**)

**38 Answer:** C: The duration, nature and mean number of attacks are pretty classic of episodic paroxysmal hemicrania, as well as the response to indomethacin (rather than cluster headache). The duration of attacks is shorter than the 30–180 minutes typical of cluster headaches.

**39 Answer B:** The most likely diagnosis is basilar migraine. The history, normal MRI brain and MR angiogram effectively exclude other possibilities offered here.

**40 Answer D:** The patient is stable and has a normal GCS. If there is evidence of raised intracranial pressure, therapies which could be considered include intravenous mannitol, barbiturate sedation and artificial hyperventilation. The treatment of choice is intravenous mannitol; steroids are not useful. Surgical intervention should only be considered if there is evidence of a cerebellar haemorrhage > 3 cm in diameter, as this is a risk for brainstem compression and ischaemia. In all other situations, surgery should only be contemplated in patients with an intermediate GCS who have had a recent presentation and are continuing to deteriorate (it should not be considered in patients who are fully rousable or totally obtunded). Surgery should be avoided if possible if the dominant hemisphere is involved. Blood pressure should only be treated if the blood pressure > 170 mmHg. Ideally, the BP is maintained at 140–160 mmHg systolic in patients with recent intracerebral haemorrhage.

**41 Answer A:** The most common symptoms of an acute cerebellar haemorrhage are severe headache and vomiting and ataxia. Patients may become comatose within hours after onset due to limited space in the posterior fossa. Pontine haemorrhage leads to rapidly deteriorating level of consciousness, impaired extraocular movement and extensive sensorimotor deficits. Basal ganglia haemorrhage leads to contralateral hemiparesis, hemisensory loss, or hemi-attention. Aphasia, especially non-fluent and impaired comprehension, is seen if haemorrhage occurs within the posterior limb of the left internal capsule. Unilateral occlusion of the anterior cerebral artery produces contralateral sensorimotor deficits mainly involving the lower extremity, with sparing of the face and hands. Occlusion of the stem of the middle cerebral artery leads to homonymous hemianopia, contralateral hemiplegia affecting the face, arm and leg, and possibly global aphasia. Posterior cerebral artery lesions produce pure hemisensory loss, visual field loss, visual agnosia and disorders of reading.

**42** **Answer B:** This patient is having recurrent episodes of anterior circulation transient ischaemic attacks (TIAs) despite being on aspirin. If aspirin alone is ineffective in preventing TIAs, then a combination of low-dose aspirin and dipyridamole modified release is recommended. There is no trial data as yet evaluating the use of clopidogrel as add on therapy to aspirin in cerebrovascular disease, although clopidogrel has been extensively evaluated in cardiovascular disease. However, clopidogrel has been shown to be an appropriate alternative for patients with a contraindication to aspirin.

**43** **Answer B:** This patient has meningitis and focal neurological signs. The CSF demonstrates a lymphocytosis in association with a raised protein count and a low glucose. The causes of a CSF lymphocytosis are shown in the Learning point at the end of this chapter. CSF immunoelectrophoresis would be useful for the diagnosis of multiple sclerosis, but this is not a likely diagnosis here. CSF pyruvate estimation is useful in the diagnosis of mitochondrial encephalopathies. The best answer here is Indian ink staining for CSF. Cryptococcal meningitis affects immunosuppressed individuals and is a recognised complication of HIV infection. The white plaques in the question suggest candida infection. (*See* **Learning point**.)

**44** **Answer A:** The combination of fatiguable proximal weakness, depressed reflexes, and autonomic dysfunction in a smoker patient suggest the diagnosis of Lambert-Eaton myaesthenic syndrome (LEMS). Positive voltage-gated calcium antibodies and EMG confirm the diagnosis; it is a paraneoplastic condition strongly associated with small cell carcinoma of the lung. He does not have anti-acetylcholine receptor antibodies, though this does not definitely mean he does not have myasthenia gravis, as around 30% of patients with this condition are anti-AChR negative. Myasthenia gravis, motor neurone disease and polymyositis do not cause autonomic impairment. Treatment is with 3,4-diaminopyridine.

**45** **Answer C:** This dentist has normal strength and notices 'twitching' or fasciculations at rest. The most likely diagnosis is benign fasciculation syndrome, a condition associated with a reduced threshold for action potentials at the neuromuscular junction, and entirely benign. Typically the patients are health professionals as they translate fasciculations to mean motor neurone disease.

46 **Answer D:** The clinical signs are compatible with a left intranuclear ophthalmoplegia. The commonest cause in a young patient is multiple sclerosis. The sensation experienced in the bath is called Lhermitte's phenomenon. The previous history of painful visual loss most likely was due to optic neuritis.

47 **Answer C:** Leber's optic atrophy usually affects young men. It causes sequential optic neuropathies within days to weeks. It is typically painless and severe. Visual acuity fails to improve. Optic neuritis is usually painful, and visual acuity improves over a matter of weeks. Giant cell arteritis affects elderly patients. Alcohol/tobacco optic neuropathies are usually chronic.

48 **Answer D:** Chalky-pale disk leads to optic atrophy. The diagnosis is anterior ischaemic optic neuropathy – arteritic or non-arteritic.

49 **Answer C:** The presentation is characteristic of acute primary closed angle glaucoma. The eyeball feels hard on palpation. It occurs in hypermetropic people with small eyeballs in whom the anterior chamber drainage angle is congenitally narrow. The acute attack begins when the iris becomes apposed to the lens and prevents the efflux of aqueous humour from the posterior chamber to the anterior chamber via the pupil. This tends to push the iris root over the trabecular meshwork, thereby blocking the drainage angle and resulting in a rise in intraocular pressure. Emergency treatment with agents to lower pressure is followed by laser iridotomy when the acute attack settles. Pilocarpine may be used in the meantime, allowing drainage to occur.

50 **Answer C:** Loss of visual acuity in this case is most consistent with ethambutol-induced optic neuritis. Ethambutol may produce optic neuritis, which decreases visual acuity and which appears to be related to dose and duration of treatment. Symptoms generally start between four months and one year after starting therapy. The effects are generally reversible when administration of ethambutol is discontinued promptly. In rare cases recovery may be delayed for one year or more, and the effect may possibly be irreversible in these cases. Although the patient has advanced HIV, with a low CD4 count and might be susceptible to CMV or toxoplasma retinitis, both of these conditions are usually associated with retinal lesions that would be visible on fundoscopy. Reduced visual acuity is not typically seen with any of the antiretrovirals listed.

51 **Answer D:** Despite the 'red-herring' of cannabis use, the diagnosis is schizophrenia, the first-rank symptoms of which are auditory hallucinations, thought disorder, features of passivity, and delusional perception.

52 **Answer C:** Pregnancy is an acknowledged cause of Wernicke's encephalopathy. Thiamine replacement would be the treatment of choice. Wernicke's encephalopathy is associated with pregnancy/hyperemesis gravidarum, as well as alcoholism.

53 **Answer E:** The most likely diagnosis again is Wernicke's encephalopathy, characterised by confusion, ataxia and gaze palsies. Intravenous thiamine should be given immediately in such situations. The commonest cause is chronic alcohol abuse.

54 **Answer E:** The presentation is oculogyric crisis, a form of drug-induced dystonia. Dopamine antagonists are well known to cause these effects. Option D would make it worse. E or benztropine would be correct answers.

55 **Answer C:** The presentation is suggestive of major depression because of the psychomotor retardation. Typical vegetative symptoms include anorexia, weight loss and insomnia, particularly early morning awakening. Psychotic symptoms such as delusions and hallucinations may occur in depression, and when they do, treatment with both an antidepressant and an antipsychotic is indicated. In alcohol-induced psychotic disorder with hallucinations, the patient may have auditory hallucinations, usually voices. The voices are characteristically maligning, reproachful or threatening. The hallucinations usually last less than a week. After the episode, most patients realise the hallucinatory nature of the symptoms. Korsakoff's psychosis is characterised by both anterograde and retrograde amnesia, with confabulation early in the course. In psychotic depression, the depression is of psychotic intensity, with delusional convictions of disease, putrefaction and poverty, contaminating others or causing evil. There may also be hallucinations, typically accusing or derogatory voices. Core symptoms of schizophrenia are delusions, hallucinations, disorganised speech, negative symptoms (e.g. blunted affect and poverty of speech) and disorganised behaviour.

56 **Answer B:** The diagnosis is neuroleptic malignant syndrome (NMS), which can occur at any time during the treatment of antipsychotic medications. Concomitant treatment with lithium or anticholinergics may increase the risk of NMS. It is manifested by fever, rigidity, altered mental status and autonomic dysfunction. Treatment includes withdrawal of the offending drug, reduction of body temperature with antipyretics. Dantrolene, bromocriptine or levodopa preparations may be beneficial.

# Learning Points

## *Question 9*

### Learning point

**Vertebral artery dissection**

Activities or events previously performed, and risk factors, which are associated with the development of vertebral artery dissection include: judo; yoga; ceiling painting; nose blowing; minor neck trauma; road traffic accident; chiropractitioner manipulation; hypertension; oral contraceptive use; tennis; golf; hairdressing; and female gender. Damage to the lateral spinothalamic and, sometimes, pyramidal tracts will cause contralateral hemianaesthesiae and upper motor neurone signs in the arm and leg. Vertebral artery dissection is a well-recognised cause of stroke in patients < 45 years and is associated with a 10% mortality rate in the acute phase. Death may occur due to intracranial dissection, brainstem infarction or subarachnoid haemorrhage. The typical clinical presentation is with severe occipital headache, followed by focal neurological signs attributable to ischaemia of brainstem or cerebellum.

Common symptoms and signs include:

Ipsilateral facial pain and/or numbness (the most common symptom)

Vertigo (very common)

Dysarthria or hoarseness (CN IX and X)

Ipsilateral limb or trunk numbness (cuneate and gracile nuclei)

Ipsilateral loss of taste (nucleus and tractus solitarius)

Hiccups

Vertigo

Nausea and vomiting

Diplopia or oscillopsia (image movement experienced with head motion)

Dysphagia (CN IX and X)

Depending upon which areas of the brain stem or cerebellum are affected, clinical signs may include:

Limb or truncal ataxia

Nystagmus

Ipsilateral Horner's syndrome (up to 1/3rd patients affected)

Ipsilateral impairment of fine touch and proprioception

Contralateral impairment of pain and thermal sensation in the extremities (i.e. spinothalamic tract)

Contralateral hemiparesis

Lateral medullary syndrome

Tongue deviation to the side of the lesion (impairment of CN XII)

Internuclear ophthalmoplegia (lesion of the medial longitudinal fasciculus)

## *Question 37*

### Learning point

**Associations of benign intracranial hypertension**

Young obese females

Pregnancy

OCP

Hypocortisolism

Hypoparathyroidism

Hypo-/Hyper-vitaminosis A

Tetracyclines

Nitrofurantoin

Nalidixic acid

Danazol

## *Question 43*

### Learning point

**CSF lymphocytosis and elevated CSF protein**

The differential diagnosis of such a CSF includes different types: infective (tuberculosis, brucellosis, listeriosis, neurosyphilis, partially treated bacterial meningitis, cerebral abscess, cryptococcal meningitis), and non-infective (CSF lymphoma, sarcoidosis, Behcet's syndrome, multiple sclerosis and disseminated CSF malignancy).

CHAPTER 11

# Endocrinology and metabolic medicine

Endocrinology and metabolic medicine questions are generally fair, as they tend to reflect what is common. Since thyroid disease is so common, a broad understanding of the clinical presentation, underlying biological mechanisms, and treatment of thyroid disease is a favourite topic. However, other topics are equally important (including tests of adrenocortical function, adrenal hypo-and hyper-functioning, hypertension, ovary and testis medicine, growth, parathyroid disease, disorders of lipid metabolism, and in particular diabetes mellitus).

## NORMAL VALUES

### Adrenal steroids

| | |
|---|---|
| Blood: | |
| serum cortisol (9 a.m.) | 200–700 nmol/L |
| serum dehydroepiandrosterone sulphate: | |
| (males) | 2–10 μmol/L |
| (females) | 3–12 μmol/L |
| Urine: | |
| cortisol | 55–250 nmol/24h |

### Anterior pituitary hormones

| | |
|---|---|
| plasma follicle stimulating hormone | 25–70 iU/L |
| plasma luteinising hormone | 25–70 iU/L |
| plasma prolactin | < 360 miU/L |

| | |
|---|---|
| plasma thyroid stimulating hormone | 0.4–5 miU/L |
| sex hormone binding globulin (SHBG) | 40–130 nmol/L |

**Thyroid and associated hormones**

| | |
|---|---|
| plasma thyroxine (T4) | 58–174 nmol/L |
| free T4 | 10–22 pmol/L |
| plasma tri-iodothyronine (T3) | 1.07–3.18 nmol/L |
| free T3 | 5–10 pmol/L |
| serum antithyroid peroxidase | < 50 iU/mL |
| serum thyroid receptor antibodies | < 10 iU/L |
| plasma parathyroid hormone | 0.9–5.4 pmol/L |
| plasma calcitonin | < 27 pmol/L |

**Sex hormones**

| | |
|---|---|
| plasma oestradiol | 130–550 pmol/L |

**Leucocyte enzymes**

| | |
|---|---|
| galactosidase A | 50–150 nmol/L |

**Pancreatic hormones**

| | |
|---|---|
| plasma 3β-hydroxybutyrate | > 1 mmol/L |
| plasma insulin | < 21 |
| C-peptide | < 0.5 |

**Urine**

| | |
|---|---|
| vanillyl mandelic acid | 5–35 μmol/24h |
| urine free metadrenaline | < 5 μmol/24h |

**Lipids and lipoproteins**

[The target levels will vary depending on the patient's overall cardiovascular risk assessment. ]

| | |
|---|---|
| serum cholesterol | < 5.2 mmol/L |
| serum LDL cholesterol | < 3.36 mmol/L |
| serum HDL cholesterol | > 1.55 mmol/L |
| fasting serum triglyceride | 0.45–1.69 mmol/L |

# Questions

## Question 1

A 26-year-old female is referred with intermittent diarrhoea for many years. She states that her weight had been steady, but describes watery motions up to six stools per day, and has also noted abdominal discomfort with bloating. She has not been aware of any blood in the motions or melaena. She describes no other medical history and denies taking any prescribed medication.

**Investigations reveal:**

| | |
|---|---|
| full blood count | normal |
| serum urea and electrolytes | normal |
| serum albumin | 39 g/L |
| serum corrected calcium | 2.2 mmol/L |
| serum alkaline phosphatase | 95 U/L |
| serum C-reactive protein | 6 mg/L |
| prothrombin time | 12 s |

What is the most likely diagnosis?

A Crohn's disease

B intestinal tuberculosis

C lactose intolerance

D laxative abuse

E microscopic colitis

## Question 2

A 25-year-old female is brought to Casualty in a London teaching hospital by her mother with a 48 hour history of severe abdominal pain and vomiting. Her mother also commented that the woman had become increasingly paranoid over the previous two weeks and felt that her line-manager was considering her dismissal. On examination, she was tachycardic at 120/min regular, BP 140/92 mmHg, cardiovascular and respiratory examinations were normal. General abdominal tenderness was noted but bowel sounds were present. Rectal examination was normal. Cranial nerves were normal, wrist extension was weak; also weak were finger extension, wrist flexion, finger flexion, and the intrinsic muscles of the hand. The biceps and supinator jerks were absent. The rest of a formal neurological examination revealed no abnormality.

**Investigations reveal:**

**Blood tests:**

| | |
|---|---|
| serum sodium | 129 mmol/L |
| serum potassium | 4.5 mmol/L |
| serum urea | 4 mmol/L |
| serum creatinine | 66 µmol/L |
| haemoglobin | 10.9 g/L |
| erythrocyte sedimentation rate | 5 mm/hour (Westergren) |
| serum C-reactive protein | 16 mg/L |

**Further tests:**

| | |
|---|---|
| **Blood film:** | normochromic and normocytic appearance |
| **Urinary dipstix:** | protein (+), urobilinogen (+++) |

What is the likely diagnosis?

A pregnancy

B familial Mediterranean fever

C acute intermittent porphyria

D systemic lupus erythematosus

E syphilis

## Question 3

A 28-year-old woman in her first pregnancy gives birth to a baby boy. The course of the pregnancy is unremarkable. From birth, the baby is noted to be lethargic, feeding poorly and vomiting frequently. On examination, he is suspected to have cataracts and this is confirmed by an ophthalmologist. He is also noted to be generally hypotonic. Over the next two weeks, his weight gain is poor and he appears increasingly irritable. He is found to have a pyrexia of 39°C, and subsequent blood cultures grow *E. coli*. He is treated with antibiotics with some improvement of his condition. There is no family history of note.

What is the most likely diagnosis in this baby?

A galactokinase deficiency
B galactosaemia
C hereditary fructose intolerance
D myotonic dystrophy
E Werdnig-Hoffman disease

## Question 4

A 24-year-old overweight woman (BMI 28 $kg/m^2$), being investigated for hirsutism and secondary amenorrhoea, had the following biochemical results:

| | |
|---|---|
| plasma oestradiol | 200 pmol/L |
| plasma luteinsing hormone | 9.0 miU/L |
| plasma follicle stimulating hormone | 2.3 miU/L |
| sex hormone binding globulin (SHBG) | 23 nmol/L |
| plasma prolactin | 800 miU/L |
| plasma testosterone | 3.4 nmol/L |
| DHEAS | 5.5 μmol/L |

What is the most likely diagnosis?

A polycystic ovary syndrome (PCOS)
B androgen-producing ovarian tumour
C congenital adrenal hyperplasia
D premature ovarian failure
E prolactinoma

## Question 5

A 25-year-old man with no medical history presented to the dermatologist with a 10 year history of progressive skin lesions located between the umbilicus and the knees. He also complained of intermittent painful episodes affecting his arms and legs which consisted of severe burning paraesthesiae. On examination, he had a blood pressure of 110/70 mmHg. There was evidence of telangiectasias affecting his penis, scrotum, thighs, buttocks and knees. He had bilateral slight corneal opacities and on slit lamp examination there was evidence of corneal atrophy.

**Investigations revealed:**

| **Blood tests:** | |
|---|---|
| full blood count | normal |
| serum sodium | 138 mmol/L |
| serum potassium | 5.2 mmol/L |
| serum urea | 11 mmol/L |
| serum creatinine | 130 μmol/L |
| **Further tests:** | |
| **Urinalysis:** | protein |
| **Skin biopsy:** | dilatation of capillaries with lipid inclusions |
| **Leucocytes:** | galactosidase A, 1.7 nmol/L |

What is the diagnosis?

A Fabry's disease

B Gaucher's disease

C erythromelalgia

D erythema gyratum

E dermatitis herpetiformis

## Question 6

An 84-year-old man is sent up to the Accident and Emergency Department by his GP. He is complaining of weakness and general malaise. He has complained of general pains in the muscles and he also has pains in his joints, particularly the elbows, wrists and knees. He lives alone in a second-floor flat. His wife died five years ago. On examination, he is edentulous, demonstrates a petechial rash prominent around hair follicles, is tender over the muscles over his limb girdles and there is mild tenderness over his elbows, wrists and knees. There are no other abnormalities to find in general examination, apart from a poorly healing wound on his right shin.

**Investigations reveal:**

| | |
|---|---|
| haemoglobin | 10.1 g/L |
| MCV | 74 fl |
| white cell count | $7.9 \times 10^9$/L (neutropils $6.3 \times 10^9$/L and lymphocytes $1.2 \times 10^9$/L) |
| platelet count | $334 \times 10^9$/L |

What is the most likely diagnosis?

A peptic ulcer

B thalassaemia trait

C scurvy

D colonic carcinoma

E idiopathic thrombocytopaenia purpura

## Question 7

A 52-year-old type 2 diabetic woman presents for her annual review. She was diagnosed with diabetes three years previously and was diagnosed with hypertension two years previously. Currently she remains on diet control alone for her diabetes and is taking bendroflumethiazine (bendrofluazide) 2.5 mg daily. There is no other past history of note. She stopped smoking five years ago and drinks approximately 5 glasses of wine weekly. On examination, she has a body mass index of 33.1 kg/m$^2$, a pulse of 88/min and a blood pressure of 160/92 mmHg. Her peripheral pulses are all present and she has a slight reduction of light touch sensation in the feet. Fundoscopy through dilated pupils reveals some hard exudates close to the macula bilaterally.

**Investigations reveal:**

| | |
|---|---|
| full blood count | normal |
| serum sodium | 141 mmol/L |
| serum potassium | 3.5 mmol/L |
| serum urea | 10.2 mmol/L |
| serum creatinine | 160 µmol/L |
| fasting plasma glucose | 12.5 mmol/L |
| HbA1c | 8.1% |

Which of the following will be the most appropriate treatment to reduce cardiovascular risk?

A insulin

B metformin

C ramipril

D reduce dietary salt

E orlistat

## Question 8

A 50-year-old male presents to the Outpatient clinic for a routine check up. He has a three year history of type II diabetes mellitus and is currently diet controlled. He takes no other medication. Examination reveals that he is obese with a BMI of 34 kg/m$^2$, his blood pressure is 180/90 mmHg and he has a pulse of 80/min regular. A check of his joint management record shows that the previous week his blood pressure was 160/90 mmHg and 170/95 mmHg. He has no evidence of any end organ damage and his pinprick sensation using a neurotip is normal.

| | |
|---|---|
| serum sodium | 136 mmol/L |
| serum potassium | 4 mmol/L |
| serum urea | 5 mmol/L |
| serum creatinine | 110 μmol/L |
| serum bicarbonate | 24 mmol/L |
| serum cholesterol | 5.4 mmol/L |
| urine albumin | 220 μmol/L |
| HbA1c | 7.4% |

Which one of these medications does not have adequate evidence for its ability to reduce cardiovascular risk?

A ACE inhibitor

B aspirin

C insulin

D metformin

E statins

## Question 9

A 23-year-old newly qualified nurse from Swansea is admitted for prolonged fasting. She originally presented to clinic with a history of episodic sweating and light-headedness which had developed over a six month period, with symptoms being entirely relieved by eating. She had developed one of these episodes whilst on the ward and a BM monitor showed a value of 2 mmol/L. She took some glucose tablets and had quickly recovered. On examination no specific abnormalities were found with a blood pressure of 118/74 mmHg, a pulse of 72/min and a BMI of 22 kg/m$^2$. She was admitted for a 72 hour fast and at 3 a.m., 16 hours into the fast, she develops typical symptoms. Her BM is measured at 2.2 mmol/L, the fast is stopped and bloods taken. The results show:

| | |
|---|---|
| plasma glucose | 1.8 mmol/L |
| plasma 3β-hydroxybutyrate | 0.5 mmol/L |
| plasma insulin | 450 pmol/L |
| C-peptide | 0.2 nmol/L |

What is the most likely diagnosis?

A adult glycogen storage disorder

B factitious hypoglycaemia due to insulin treatment

C factitious hypoglycaemia due to sulphonylurea treatment

D insulinoma

E non-islet cell tumour

## Question 10

A 44-year-old male attends for a health check at a mobile cardiovascular risk assessment clinic. He takes no medication but leads a sedentary lifestyle. He is a non-smoker and family history reveals that his father had an myocardial infarction at 60 years old.

**Investigations reveal:**

| | |
|---|---|
| fasting total cholesterol | 5.0 mmol/L |
| fasting triglycerides | 4.0 mmol/L |
| normal full blood count and MCV | |

Which of the following is the commonest cause of these results?

A alcohol

B diabetes mellitus

C drug therapy

D familial hyperlipidaemia

E obesity

## Question 11

A 68-year-old estate agent was admitted with nausea and general malaise. Over the last two weeks, since returning from holiday in Spain, he had become increasingly fatigued and breathless. The only other symptoms of note were a 3 month history of poor appetite and an 8 kg weight loss. He was receiving thyroxine 100 mcg daily, having been diagnosed with hypothyroidism by his GP nine years previously. He was a smoker of 5 cigarettes per day and had drunk more alcohol than usual whilst on holiday, but usually drank about 12 units of alcohol a week. On examination, he was sun-tanned, slightly confused, appeared dehydrated and had a pulse of 92/min regular, a temperature of 37.2°C with a blood pressure of standing 112/80 mmHg with a significant postural drop. Cardiovascular and respiratory examination were unremarkable. He had a slight liver edge on palpation and neurological examination was normal.

**Investigations revealed:**

| | |
|---|---|
| BM | 2.4 |
| serum sodium | 129 mmol/L |
| serum potassium | 5.2 mmol/L |
| serum corrected calcium | 2.73 mmol/L |
| serum standard bicarbonate | 15 mmol/L |
| serum urea | 22 mmol/L |
| plasma TSH | 6 miU/L |

Which of the following is the most likely diagnosis?

A bronchogenic carcinoma with syndrome of inappropriate ADH secretion

B hypoadrenalism

C hypothyroidism

D primary hyperparathyroidism

E sarcoidosis

## Question 12

A 24-year-old woman presented with increasingly frequent episodes of hypoglycaemia. She had well controlled type 1 diabetes mellitus for eight years.

**Investigations revealed:**

| | |
|---|---|
| serum sodium | 128 mmol/L |
| serum potassium | 4.5 mmol/L |
| serum urea | 6.8 mmol/L |
| serum creatinine | 70 µmol/L |
| plasma glucose | 4.2 mmol/L |
| C-peptide | normal |

What is the next best investigation?

A urinary β-HCG level

B fasting C-peptide level

C short synacthen test

D serum renin level

E chest x-ray

## Question 13

A 25-year-old female of Bangladeshi origin presents with weight loss and fatigue of approximately four months duration. She arrived back in the UK three months ago after spending one year in Bangladesh with her parents' family, and returned due to ill health. She has otherwise been quite well with no other medical history, has two children, is a non-smoker and drinks no alcohol. On examination, she is thin with a BMI of 20 kg/m$^2$, has obvious pigmentation of the palmar creases, has pigmentation of the buccal mucosa, a pulse of 77/min (sinus rhythm), and a lying blood pressure of 100/62 mmHg. No other abnormalities are evident on examination.

**Investigations reveal:**

| | |
|---|---|
| haemoglobin | 11.2 g/L |
| MCV | 78 fL |
| white cell count | 9.0 × 10$^9$/L |
| serum sodium | 130 mmol/L |
| serum potassium | 5 mmol/L |
| serum urea | 7.8 mmol/L |
| serum creatinine | 110 μmol/L |
| plasma glucose | 5 mmol/L |
| erythrocyte sedimentation rate | 60 mm/hr (Westergren) |
| 9 a.m. serum cortisol | 90 nmol/L |

Which of the following would be the most appropriate investigation for this patient?

A CT abdomen

B CT pituitary

C CT thorax

D PA chest x-ray

E radiolabelled white cell scan

## Question 14

A 17-year-old female presents with a two day history of vomiting, general lethargy and giddiness. Over the last six months she had lost 5 kg in weight, had a reduced appetite and had been feeling increasingly lethargic. Friends note that she has been reading women's magazines regularly, and has been talking more often about the importance of looking thin. She has no past medical history of note, is a non-smoker and takes the combined oral contraceptive pill. Her eldest brother was well and there was a family history of thyroid disease, with both her mother and her maternal grandmother taking thyroxine. On examination, she was comfortable at rest, appeared slightly dehydrated, was apyrexial, had a body mass index of 18.5 kg/m$^2$ and oxygen saturations on air of 99%. Her blood pressure was 102/64 mmHg and fell to 86/60 mmHg on standing. Her pulse was 90/min regular and auscultation of the heart and chest were normal. No abnormalities were detected on abdominal or CNS examination.

**Investigations reveal:**

| | |
|---|---|
| haemoglobin | 10.5 g/L |
| MCV | 86 fL |
| white cell count | 8.8 × 10$^9$/L |
| neutrophils | 4.4 × 10$^9$/L |
| lymphocytes | 2.8 × 10$^9$/L |
| eosinophils | 0.8 × 10$^9$/L |
| serum sodium | 130 mmol/L |
| serum potassium | 5.8 mmol/L |
| serum urea | 12.8 mmol/L |
| serum creatinine | 135 μmol/L |
| plasma glucose | 3.8 mmol/L |
| free T4 | 8.8 pmol/L |
| TSH | 1.2 miU/L |
| **Urinalysis:** | ketones (+) |

Which of the following is the most appropriate initial investigation?

A adrenal autoantibodies

B CT scan of the adrenals

C MRI scan of the pituitary

D short synacthen test

E neuropsychiatric assessment

## Question 15

A 70-year-old retired office clerk is admitted with confusion and dehydration. Her relatives claim that she has been deteriorating over the last couple of months. They have noticed that lately she has become incontinent of urine and that she has become more withdrawn and depressed. She personally has not noticed any changes, apart from non-specific abdominal pain, and that she has become rather more thirsty than usual. Her past medical history is unremarkable except for hypertension diagnosed three years ago originally attributed as a 'white-coat effect', but for which she now takes bendrofluazide (bendroflumethiazine) 2.5 mg daily and amlodipine 10 mg daily. On examination she is confused but alert. She knows her name and address but does not know where she is. She appears clinically dehydrated, with a pulse of 110/min regular, a blood pressure of 194/88 mmHg and is apyrexial. Examination of the cardiovascular system, abdomen and chest are all normal apart from mild tenderness in the upper middle quadrant. No goitre is palpable but breast examination reveals generally nodular breasts.

**Investigations reveal:**

| | |
|---|---|
| haemoglobin | 13.2 g/L |
| white cell count | 9.0 × $10^9$/L |
| serum sodium | 146 mmol/L |
| serum potassium | 3.3 mmol/L |
| serum urea | 12.1 mmol/L |
| serum creatinine | 250 µmol/L |
| serum calcium | 4.2 mmol/L |
| serum phosphate | 0.8 mmol/L |
| plasma parathyroid hormone | 121 nmol/L |

What is the most likely diagnosis?

A multiple myeloma

B multiple bony metastases

C occult cancer with ectopic PTH-related peptide secretion

D parathyroid adenoma

E parathyroid carcinoma

## Question 16

A 17-year-old boy is brought into Casualty unconscious. His mother said that he had recently become aggressive and irrational, and had recently smashed several windows in the house for no apparent reason. She mentioned that he had been perfectly well until his father died after an emergency operation for 'burst ulcer' a year beforehand. Since then his personality had changed. He had become increasingly irritable and aggressive and had taken to eating sweets and snacks during the day. For this reason, he had put on 30 kg over the past year. He had had a kidney stone removed two years previously, and had a neck operation shortly afterwards. On examination, he was unrousable with a flaccid paresis. He was unresponsive to pain with a GCS of 7 (localising to pain). Reflexes were normal. Pupils were dilated, but responsive to light. Pulse was 140/min regular, blood pressure 160/90, JVP normal. Heart sounds were normal. Respiratory examination was unremarkable. Abdominal examination was normal.

What is the most likely diagnosis?

A polyglandular autoimmune syndrome type 1 (APECED)

B polyglandular autoimmune syndrome type 2 (Schmidt's syndrome)

C multiple endocrine neoplasia type 1

D multiple endocrine neoplasia type 2

E none of the above

## Question 17

A 25-year-old male is referred with hypertension, agitation and sweats of approximately six months' duration. He has no specific family history of note, smokes 10 cigarettes per day and drinks little alcohol. Medication prescribed by his GP for hypertension includes bendroflumethiazine (bendrofluazide) 2.5 mg/d and ramipril 10 mg per day. His blood pressure on examination was 176/94 mmHg and he has a BMI of 23.5 kg/m$^2$. MRI scan of the abdomen revealed a 3.5 cm mass in the right adrenal gland.

**Further investigations reveal:**

| | |
|---|---|
| urine free metadrenaline | 12 μmol/a day |
| fasting plasma calcitonin | 100 ng/L |

Based on this information, what other diagnosis is likely to be associated with this man's condition?

A acoustic neuroma

B gastrinoma

C hyperparathyroidism

D insulinoma

E prolactinoma

## Question 18

A 26-year-old man underwent total parathyroidectomy for hyperparathyroidism secondary to parathyroid hyperplasia. During surgery, he had a blood pressure of 190/110 mmHg. His father also had a past history of hyperparathyroidism.

What is the best medication for his hypertension?

A nifedipine

B hydralazine

C lisinopril

D atenolol

E labetalol

## Question 19

A 45-year-old female presents with depression, constipation, polyuria and thirst. Over the last six months she has become increasingly aware of tiredness and arthralgia since being diagnosed with hypertension and has been treated with bendroflumethiazine (bendrofluazide) 2.5 mg daily. Physical examination proves to be entirely normal except for a blood pressure of 162/94 mmHg.

**Investigations reveal:**

| | |
|---|---|
| haemoglobin | 14.4 g/L |
| white cell count | 7.1 × $10^9$/L |
| platelet count | 200 × $10^9$/L |
| serum sodium | 148 mmol/L |
| serum potassium | 4.2 mmol/L |
| serum chloride | 105 mmol/L |
| serum bicarbonate | 28 mmol/L |
| serum urea | 8 mmol/L |
| serum creatinine | 105 µmol/L |
| serum corrected calcium | 3.2 mmol/L |
| serum total bilirubin | 16 µmol/L |
| serum alanine aminotransferase | 10 U/L |
| serum alkaline phosphatase | 130 U/L |
| plasma parathyroid hormone | 17 pmol/L |

Which of the following is the most appropriate initial therapy?

A calcitonin

B frusemide (furosemide)

C intravenous normal saline

D pamidronate

E steroids

## Question 20

These results are from a 78-year-old man with a short history of peri-oral and peripheral tingling and mild confusion. He had been treated for two years with Zoladex for metastatic prostatic carcinoma.

**Investigations revealed:**

| | |
|---|---|
| serum sodium | 141 mmol/L |
| serum potassium | 4.1 mmol/L |
| serum creatinine | 156 µmol/L |
| serum corrected calcium | 1.4 mmol/L |
| serum alkaline phosphatase | 20 ng/mL |
| serum prostate-specific antigen | 10 µg/L |

The most likely diagnosis is:

A hypoparathyroidism

B osteomalacia

C Paget's disease

D oncogenic phosphaturia

E hungry bone syndrome

## Question 21

A 52-year-old woman is referred by an orthopaedic surgeon for advice following a Colle's fracture eight weeks ago. At the time of her fracture, the radiologist had reported 'significant osteopenia'. A dual-energy x-ray absorptiometry (DEXA) scan was carried out and her *T*-score was –2.6 at the hip and –1.9 at the lumbar spine. She smokes approximately 15 cigarettes per day and has a body mass index of 21 kg/m$^2$. She has been post-menopausal for two years, is unaware of any menopausal symptoms and has had a benign breast lump removed 18 months ago. She is currently taking aspirin, atenolol and glyceryl trinitrate (GTN) spray for her angina, which she only uses occasionally.

What would be the most appropriate treatment?

A calcitonin

B calcium and vitamin D supplements

C hormone replacement therapy

D raloxifene

E risedronate

## Question 22

A 42-year-old female presented with acute back pain after lifting a chair from her office to the storage cupboard. The pain is described as intense, increasing upon movement, and radiating bilaterally around the hypochondrium. Upon questioning she denied previous fractures, but admitted to a gradual loss of height (5 cm from her young adult height) and occasional self-limiting back pain. Past medical history included spontaneous menopause at the age of 37. She had never taken any regular medications in the past, calcium or vitamin D supplements. Examination revealed a thin woman who had a dorsal hyperkyphosis. Severe back pain was elicited on movement and local percussion. Investigations (which involved bone mineral density (BMD), assessed by dual-energy x-ray absorptiometry (DEXA) at the hip and the lumbar spine (L1–L4)) showed a BMD *T*-score at lumber spine: –3.0 and a BMD *T*-score at total hip: –2.8.

What is the diagnosis?

A osteopaenia

B osteomalacia secondary to vitamin D or calcium deficiency

C post-menopausal osteoporotic vertebral fractures

D senile osteoporosis

E vertebral fractures secondary to malignant infiltration

## Question 23

A 74-year-old woman with a previous hip fracture was referred to the endocrine clinic with a suspected diagnosis of osteoporosis. She also complained of increasing thirst and nocturia. Urinalysis was normal. Baseline tests performed by her GP showed: serum calcium 3.5 mmol/L, serum phosphate 0.6 mmol/L, serum alkaline phosphatase 220 U/L, serum urea 7 mmol/L, serum creatinine 123 µmol/L, glucose 6 mmol/L and erythrocyte sedimentation rate 23 mm/hr.

The most likely diagnosis is:

A primary hyperparathyroidism

B hypercalcaemia of malignancy

C Paget's disease of bone

D secondary hyperparathyroidism

E familial hypocalciuric hypercalcaemia

## Question 24

A 29-year-old woman is admitted for the investigation of lethargy and weakness. She had a past history of depression and had drunk close to ten bottles of sparkling wine per week for the last three years. On admission, she was taking amitriptyline. On examination, she was plethoric and obese, BP 160/100 mmHg. Serum cortisol measured at 9 a.m. was 867 nmol/L. After 0.5 mg of dexamethasone six hourly for 48 hours, 9 a.m. serum cortisol was measured at 750 nmol/L. After 2 mg of dexamethasone 6 hourly for 48 hours, 9 a.m. serum cortisol 310 nmol/L. Twenty-four hours later 9 a.m. serum cortisol was 120 nmol/L.

The most likely diagnosis is:

A primary depression

B ectopic ACTH secretion

C Cushing's disease

D alcoholic pseudo-cushing's syndrome

E adrenal adenoma

## Question 25

A 45-year-old male presents with some two years' history of impotence and reduced shaving frequency. These symptoms have evolved over this period of time, he is unaware of any erections whatsoever and has no libido. He also is aware that he shaves just once weekly, whereas previously he was shaving daily. Together with these symptoms he has also been feeling rather lethargic, with reduced energy and is aware of vague joint aches. He takes no medication and has otherwise been well except for an appendicectomy at the age of 20. He drinks approximately 20 units of alcohol weekly and smokes around five cigarettes daily. He is married but has no children. On examination, he appears slightly pigmented, has gynaecomastia and a fine skin with scant facial, pubic and axillary hair. Examination of the testes reveal testicular size of approximately 15 mL bilaterally and no masses are felt. Examination of the cardiovascular, respiratory and abdominal systems is normal. No abnormalities are noted on joint movements with a full range of movement.

**Investigations reveal:**

| | |
|---|---|
| plasma prolactin | 370 miU/L |
| free T4 | 12.8 nmol/L |
| plasma thyroid stimulating hormone | 2.1 miU/L |
| serum testosterone | 4 nmol/L |
| plasma luteinising hormone | 1.2 iU/L |
| plasma follice stimulating hormone | 1.3 iU/L |
| serum aspartate aminotransferase | 40 iU/L |
| serum alanine aminotransferase | 60 iU/L |
| serum alkaline phosphatase | 100 U/L |

Which of the following is the most important initial investigation?

A transferrin saturation

B karyotype

C MRI of the pituitary

D short synacthen test

E ultrasound of the testes

## Question 26

A 62-year-old male is referred with impotence. He was diagnosed with diabetes mellitus 10 years ago and was initially treated with diet but has required metformin over the last three years. Five years previously, he underwent a left hip replacement. Over the last two years he has been aware of deteriorating erectile dysfunction and is now totally impotent. He shaves daily and has not been aware of any change in body hair. He is a non-smoker and drinks approximately ten units of alcohol weekly. There was no history of buttock claudication. Examination reveals an obese male with a blood pressure of 146/88 mmHg, who had normal secondary sexual characteristics. Testicular examination reveals normal testes of approximately 15 mL in volume. There are no abnormalities on cardiovascular, respiratory or abdominal examinations, including normal femoral pulses.

**Investigations reveal:**

| | |
|---|---|
| haemoglobin | 14.2 g/L |
| white cell count | 9.0 × $10^9$/L |
| platelet count | 190 × $10^9$/L |
| serum sodium | 145 mmol/L |
| serum potassium | 4.5 mmol/L |
| serum urea | 7.2 mmol/L |
| serum creatinine | 110 µmol/L |
| serum alkaline phosphatase | 88 U/L |
| serum aspirate aminotransferase | 40 iU/L |
| serum gamma glutaryltransferase | 40 iU/L |
| HbA1c | 7.8% |
| fasting plasma glucose | 7.8 nmol/L |
| plasma total testosterone | 7.1 nmol/L |
| plasma follicle stimulating hormone | 4.1 iU/L |
| plasma luteinsing hormone | 5.1 iU/L |

What is the next best initial investigation?

A serum ferritin

B MRI scan of the head

C oestradiol concentration

D prolactin concentration

E ultrasound of the testes

## Question 27

A 29-year-old woman complained of increasing lethargy and weight gain over the previous six months. Her only medication consisted of the combined oral contraceptive pill. Her GP performed the following blood tests and asked for advice regarding further management:

| | |
|---|---|
| free T4 | 15.0 pmol/L |
| plasma thyroid stimulating hormone | 10 miU/L |

The most likely diagnosis is:

A subclinical hypothyroidism

B TSH-oma

C exogenous thyroxine abuse

D combined oral contraceptive pill

E thyroid hormone resistance syndrome

## Question 28

A 15-year-old girl complained of anxiety and excessive sweating. She was not taking any medication.

**Investigations revealed:**

| | |
|---|---|
| plasma thyroid stimulating hormone | 0.9 miU/L |
| free T4 | 16 pmol/L |
| total T4 | 180 nmol/L |
| free T3 | 8.2 pmol/L |
| total T3 | 3.3 nmol/L |

Which one of the diagnoses below are these results most compatible with?

A factitious thyrotoxicosis

B familial dysalbuminaemic hyperthyroxinaemia

C pregnancy

D sick euthyroid syndrome

E thyrotoxicosis

## Question 29

A 30-year-old female presents with general tiredness and poor appetite. She has found increasing difficulty coping at home, being particularly tired since the birth of her son two months previously. She has one other child, a girl aged three. Both pregnancies were uneventful, although she required iron supplements for anaemia during both pregnancies. She has been breast feeding quite normally and her son is quite well. There is nil of note in her past history and she takes no regular medication. There is no family history of note. On examination, she has a BMI of 24 kg/m$^2$, a pulse of 96/min and a blood pressure of 124/70 mmHg. She has a mild lid-lag, but no other ocular signs. A small palpable smooth non-tender goitre is palpable, but no bruit is audible. She has a slight tremor of her outstretched hands. Cardiovascular, respiratory and abdominal examinations are normal.

| | |
|---|---|
| haemoglobin | 11.2 g/L |
| erythrocyte sedimentation rate | 21 mm/hr (Westergren) |
| serum sodium | 136 mmol/L |
| serum potassium | 3.7 mmol/L |
| serum urea | 5.2 mmol/L |
| serum creatinine | 70 µmol/L |
| random plasma glucose | 5.2 nmol/L |
| plasma T4 | 28.2 nmol/L |
| plasma T3 | 6.8 nmol/L |
| plasma thyroid stimulating hormone | 0.05 miU/L |
| anti-thyroid peroxidase antibodies | 400 iU/L |

What is the most likely diagnosis?

A De Quervain's thyroiditis

B Graves' disease

C Hashimoto's thyrotoxicosis

D post-partum thyroiditis

E toxic nodular goitre

## Question 30

A 27-year-old female is referred by her GP being 10 weeks pregnant. Three months ago she was diagnosed with thyrotoxicosis with an elevated T4 concentration and suppressed TSH concentration. At that stage her GP started her on carbimazole. At presentation she has a pulse of 90/min (irregularly irregular), a fine tremor and lid lag. Blood pressure is 118/80 mmHg and she has a palpable goitre.

From the following select the most appropriate treatment for this patient?

**A** continue carbimazole

**B** radioactive iodine

**C** stop all drugs during pregnancy

**D** switch to propylthiouracil

**E** thyroidectomy

# Answers to Chapter 11: Endocrinology and metabolic medicine

These solutions aim to provide the reason(s) for the right answer, and also the reason(s) for the wrong answers being excluded.

1 **Answer D:** All her parameters are normal, except for her calcium, which is at the lower limit of normal. Calcium in the gut normally gets absorbed in the ileum and to a lesser extent in the jejunum and duodenum; laxative abuse causes lower bowel hurry, causing decreased absorption of calcium. Also, hpomagnesemia associated with laxative abuse can result in hypocalcemia. Lactose intolerance is unlikely because of the duration and age. Any form of colitis and other malabsorption syndromes such as ileocaecal TB causes raised C-reactive protein and decreased serum albumin, with other blood abnormalities such as anaemia.

2 **Answer C:** Acute intermittent porphyria is the most likely diagnosis. This is an autosomal dominant disorder caused by a defect in porphobilinogen deaminase activity. Many cases exist in latent form, but in manifest cases it is more frequently seen in women. The estimated prevalence of the disorder is 5–10 cases per 100 000 population. The latent form of the disease may exist indefinitely, but certain drugs, infections, and excessive dieting (starvation) can precipitate attacks. The most common drugs are sulphonamides and barbiturates (often seen when giving phenobarbital for pain relief with dental surgery). In an acute attack the neurological dysfunction can involve any portion of the nervous system. It is believed that an imbalance in the autonomic innervation of the gut leads to abdominal pain, which is commonly associated with the attack. If peripheral neuropathy, such as pain in the back and legs or parathesias, occurs, it is almost always preceded by abdominal pain. Complete flaccid paralysis can develop over a few days. Other autonomic neuropathies that may be seen are sweating, vascular spasm, labile hypertension, and sinus tachycardia. A grave sign is the development of respiratory paralysis and in very severe attacks patients are unable to speak, breathe, or swallow. Central nervous dysfunction can be seen as well with hallucinations, seizures, coma, bulbar paralysis, hypothalamic dysfunction, or cerebellar and basal ganglion involvement.

3 **Answer B:** Galactosaemia is an autosomal recessive inherited disease caused by a deficiency of the enzyme galactose-1-phosphate uridyltransferase which catalyses the reaction of galactose-1-phosphate to uridyl diphosphogalactose. Infants often become symptomatic during the early neonatal interval after dietary exposure to lactose- or galactose-containing foods. The classic clinical features are poor feeding, lethargy, failure to thrive, vomiting, hypoglycaemia, cataracts (which can occur from early life), liver dysfunction and/or

hepatomegaly, bleeding from coagulopathy and the predisposition to *E. coli* sepsis. In galactokinase deficiency, the sole clinical manifestation is cataracts, which can occur at any age. Hereditary fructose intolerance is associated with a defect in the enzyme fructose bisphosphate aldolase and is characterised by severe hypoglycaemia, vomiting, seizures, aversion to fruits, failure to thrive, liver disease and renal tubular disease. Cataracts only develop in later life in myotonic dystrophy. Werdnig-Hoffmann disease or spinal muscular atrophy type I is associated with severe hypotonia, respiratory distress, limb and bulbar muscle weakness.

4 **Answer A:** The diagnosis is PCOS. The biochemical features of this syndrome include: high LH:FSH ratio in half to two thirds of patients, high testosterone (<5 nmol/L), high/detectable oestradiol, reduced SHBG if overweight, and normal DHEAS. The treatment plan depends on the problem and includes weight reduction, if obese, to encourage insulin sensitisation, COCP (dianette is often the first choice), spironolactone, finasteride or cryproterone acetate (with adequate contraception due to teratogenicity). Metformin is a useful treatment option.

5 **Answer A:** Fabry's disease is a rare X-linked disorder in which females are asymptomatic or mildly symptomatic carriers and males exhibit the full blown disorder. There is a defect in the lysosomal enzyme galactosidase A leading to glycolipid deposition in the skin, bones, kidneys, brain, heart and ocular tissues. This condition often presents in childhood but sometimes it may present as late as the second decade. The diagnosis is suggested by cutaneous lesions (telangiectasia) located usually in a bathing trunk distribution ('angiokeratoma corporis diffusum') at the umbilicus, penis, scrotum, buttocks, hips and thighs. There is reduced sweating and paraesthesiae affecting the hands and feet with burning pain in the extremities. Patients may complain of diarrhoea or abdominal pain; ocular disorders occur in more than 80%, including lens opacities and corneal atrophy (although the retina and conjunctiva may be affected). There may be renal involvement, which manifests with proteinuria and hypertension. Patients may suffer from angina, myocardial infarction, cardiomyopathy (both hypertrophic and dilated) and cerebral disorders such as seizures and hemiplegia have been reported. Diagnosis is made by demonstrating a deficiency of $\alpha$-galactosidase A in leucocytes and skin or bone biopsy. Treatment requires a multi-disciplinary approach and consists of pain relief with carbamazepine/phenytoin or low dose opiate, renal dialysis or transplant and pulsed dye laser therapy for cutaneous lesions.

6 **Answer C:** There are a number of features that hint at an underlying nutritional disorder. He is a widower, and lives on a second-floor flat, which makes it difficult for him to get out. A number of the features suggest a possible diagnosis of scurvy from vitamin C deficiency. Body stores of vitamin C are

sufficient to last two or three months. The rash, muscle and joint pains and tenderness, poor wound healing and microcytic anaemia are all features of scurvy. The classic features of bleeding from the gums would not be present in an edentulous patient.

7 **Answer C:** The most appropriate treatment to reduce her cardiovascular risk should focus on adequate blood pressure control, supported by evidence from the UK Prospective Diabetes Study (UKPDS), which showed greater reductions in cardiovascular risk with BP control as compared with no overall reduction in cardiovascular mortality in patients with tight glycaemic control on insulin or sulphonylureas. Similarly, the Heart Outcomes Prevention Evaluation (HOPE) study demonstrated that the addition of the ACE inhibitor, ramipril, may produce even greater benefit in subjects at high cardiovascular risk. In this patient the addition of ramipril with bendrofluazide would be logical. Regular serum urea and electrolyte monitoring is very important after initiation of treatment with an ACE inhibitor. Although metformin would be expected to reduce cardiovascular risk in obese type 2 diabetics, the drug would be relatively contraindicated in this patient whose serum creatinine exceeds 150 µmol/L. Good glycaemic control also helps in reducing the risk of microvascular complications. Weight reduction has itself not been shown to reduce cardiovascular risk and as yet no studies have demonstrated this with orlistat. ACE inhibitors also have a beneficial effect on retinopathy and nephropathy, and the patient needs to have regular review for that.

8 **Answer C:** This man is an obese type II diabetic, with fair diabetic control, raised cholesterol, hypertension, and microalbuminuria. Thus we are looking at primary prevention of a cardiac event in this patient. He is at high risk of a cardiovascular event. Various studies provide evidence for primary prevention of a cardiac event with statin treatment. In the HOPE study, ramipril has been shown to lower cardiovascular risk in patients with two CV risk factors, as well as in diabetics, independently of BP lowering. In the HOT study, to name one of many, aspirin has been shown to lower the risk of CV events in high risk individuals with diabetes. Evidence from UKPDS shows that treatment of overweight, diabetic patients with metformin lowers the relative risk of myocardial infarction by 40%, with respect to treatment with sulphonylureas or insulin. There is no evidence that commencing T2Ds on insulin lowers the risk of MI, even if the HbA1c improves. However, DIGAMI showed risk reduction of sliding scale insulin, followed by subcutaneous insulin in patients with an MI (secondary prevention).

9 **Answer B:** This patient has developed hypoglycaemia with suppression of her 3β-Hydroxybutyrate (a ketone), elevated insulin, yet suppressed C-peptide. This would suggest that there is insulin-induced hypoglycaemia

and, as C-peptide is suppressed, indicates exogenous administration of insulin. Sulphonylureas would produce raised insulin and C-peptides and could be assessed in suspicious cases by measuring a sulphonylurea concentration. Again, insulinoma would be associated with proportionately elevated insulin and C-peptide. (*See* **Learning point**.)

10 **Answer E:** The commonest cause of a mild hypertriglyceridaemia is obesity secondary to a reduced efficacy of lipoprotein lipase activity and overproduction of VLDL. Obesity (defined as a BMI above 30) is present in approximately 20% of subjects in the UK and rising, and hence this is why it is the commonest cause of hyperlipidaemia. Alcohol is probably a close second. Other secondary causes of hypertriglyceridaemia include pregnancy, hypothyroidism, diuretics and pancreatitis.

11 **Answer B:** This estate agent has a three month history of weight loss, anorexia and fatigue. He has recently returned from Spain, but this is a distractor (as is his occupation). No really obvious features are present on examination. The investigations show hyponatraemia, hyperkalaemia, uraemia, hypercalcaemia, low bicarbonate and slightly elevated TSH, which suggest the diagnosis of hypoadrenalism. In addition, eosinophilia and lymphocytosis are commonly seen. He is known to have an autoimmune disease – hypothyroidism and a diagnosis of Addison's disease are suggested. Slight elevation of TSH and a mild hypercalcaemia are typical of hypoadrenalism. Bronchogenic carcinoma with SIADH would be expected to produce a hyponatraemia, but with normal potassium and serum urea. The patient's symptoms do not fit with hypothyroidism (weight loss) and the uraemia and hypercalcaemia would not be expected. Although sarcoidosis may produce the hypercalcaemia, the hyponatraemia would not be a typical finding and respiratory signs may be expected. Primary hyperparathyroidism would not produce such problems with such a calcium concentration.

12 **Answer C:** The reduced requirement for insulin and the low sodium are suggestive of Addison's disease (Schmidt's syndrome). However, hypoglycaemic attacks are also seen early in pregnancy, especially in those patients with hyperemesis gravidarum, coeliac disease, Graves' disease.

13 **Answer A:** This young woman presents after returning from a long period in Bangladesh with weight loss and lethargy. Her results are highly suggestive of a primary adrenal failure (pigmentation indicating elevated ACTH, hence primary adrenal dysfunction), low sodium, low BP and the low random cortisol. In this case, with the high erythrocyte sedimentation rate, tuberculous adrenalitis should be considered in the differential diagnosis, but also Addison's disease is still a possibility. The most appropriate initial investigation would be confirmation of hypoadrenalism with a short synacthen test. From the list above a CT adrenals would be logical and absence/shrinkage or

enlargement of the adrenals may be seen. Although a chest x-ray would be an appropriate initial investigation, the results from this may be normal despite the possibility of tuberculosis.

**14** **Answer D:** The salient features in this young patient's case are the long standing asthenia with weight loss and the sudden episode of vomiting. She appears clinically dehydrated, as demonstrated by the postural hypotension but her results reveal hyponatraemia, hyperkalaemia and hyperuricaemia. Her full blood count shows an eosinophilia. The most likely diagnosis is acute hypoadrenalism probably due to Addison's disease, in view of the strong family history of autoimmune disease. The diagnosis should be confirmed with a short synacthen test and a cortisol response less than 550 nmol/L is confirmatory. Abnormal thyroid function tests with low T4 and normal TSH are quite commonly associated with Addison's and do not reflect secondary hypothyroidism but sick euthyroidism. Thyroxine replacement must not be given to these patients as it can exacerbate the adrenal crisis. The TFTs will normalise with hydrocortisone therapy. Even if this were hypopituitarism an MRI of the pituitary would not diagnose hypoadrenalism and again this could be confirmed with a short synacthen test.

**15** **Answer E:** This patient has grossly elevated calcium and in the context of the extremely high PTH concentration, a diagnosis of parathyroid carcinoma should be considered. Parathyroid cancer is rare and the only feature that may make you suspicious of a cancer rather than adenoma is the grossly elevated PTH. This is not ectopic PTH-related peptide secretion, as PTH would be expected to be low with ectopic PTH-related peptide secretion and the latter does not cross-react with the standard PTH assay.

**16** **Answer C:** This patient most likely has multiple endocrine neoplasia type 1. The features of this syndrome are parathyroid adenomas (hypercalcaemia), pituitary tumours (including prolactinomas, somatotrophinomas, corticotrophinomas), and pancreatic tumours (including insulinomas, gastrinomas, glucagonomas, and VIPomas).

**17** **Answer C:** This patient has features of type 2 multiple endocrine neoplasia, as evidenced by phaeochromocytoma and medullary cell thyroid neoplasia, and is associated with hyperparathyroidism. MEN type 1 is associated with pancreatic and pituitary neoplasia. MEN type 2 is usually autosomal dominant but in this patient's case there appears to be a spontaneous mutation, as there is no family history of note. It is important to investigate phaeochromocytoma in the young for potential precipitating disorders such as neurofibromatosis, MEN and Von Hippel-Lindau syndrome.

**18** **Answer E:** Familial hyperparathyroidism and raised blood pressure may be unrelated, but type 2 MEN should again be considered here. In this respect, consider phaeochromocytoma. The treatment of hypertension in patients with phaeochromocytoma involves combined alpha and beta blockade. Labetalol has both α- and β-blocking properties. Pure beta-blockers may result in hypertensive crisis, due to unopposed α-blockade. The most conventional elective medical treatment is blockade with phenoxybenzamine then β-blockade. Because of volume depletion, patients often require a lot of filling.

19 **Answer C:** This patient has primary hyperparathyroidism and the hypercalcaemia should initially be treated with intravenous normal saline. She is dehydrated and requires appropriate fluid replacement. Once corrected, the patient could then be offered surgery as the most appropriate therapeutic option. Calcitonin is reserved for severe hypercalcaemia such as sarcoidosis, where, however, the effects of treatment tend to be transient. Pamidronate is effective at reducing calcium over a couple of days but it is important to first ensure that the patient is adequately hydrated. Steroids are effective in certain types of hypercalcaemia – sarcoid – but are ineffective in primary hyperparathyroidism. Frusemide (furosemide) is often used to induce a hypercalciuria in severe hypercalcaemia once the patient has been adequately rehydrated. On the other hand, bendrofluazide reduces calcium loss in the urine, thereby raising serum calcium.

20 **Answer E:** 'Hungry bone syndrome' would fit the history and investigations. While hypercalcaemia is a commonly encountered paraneoplastic manifestation, hypocalcaemia is rare. A malignant neoplasm with skeletal deposits resulting in hypocalcaemia and osteomalacia would appear to be an intriguing paradox. Approximately 60 cases have been described wherein a tumour has been clearly documented as the cause of osteomalacia. Most of these tumours were benign and the patients usually presented with classical symptoms of osteomalacia, namely: bone pain, proximal weakness and even genu valgus that resolved with resection of the neoplasia. The exact pathogenic mechanism of oncogenic osteomalacia has been a point of contention since its initial description, and it has been recently suggested that there is FGF23 secretion by the tumour, leading to increased renal phosphate leak. Early investigators proposed the increased skeletal avidity ('hungry bone', 'calcium sink') theory in which the rapid skeletal accretion of calcium by the osteoblastic metastases was believed to be responsible for the hypocalcaemia.

21 **Answer E:** Bisphosphonates (e.g. alendronate and risedronate) act as potent inhibitors of bone resorption by decreasing osteoclast recruitment, activity, and life span. Treatment with bisphosphonates has been shown to significantly increase bone mineral density (BMD) in osteoporotic patients and thus to reduce fractures. Problems with adverse effects (mainly GI upset) can be reduced by a weekly administration of bisphosphonates. It is the drug of

choice in this situation. Calcium and vitamin D supplements are more likely to benefit women who are > 5 years post-menopause, as their intake is likely to be low. Postmenopausal women who wish to reduce the risk of osteoporosis should consume 1000–1500 mg of elemental calcium and 400–800 iU of vitamin D daily, ideally through calcium-containing foods. Excessive intake of calcium and vitamin D may cause adverse effects such as hypercalcaemia hypercalciuria. The use of hormone replacement therapy (HRT) is controversial and should be reserved for those with menopausal symptoms and without overt cardiovascular disease, as studies suggest increased cardiovascular risk, although it is still a good agent in preventing fractures. (Breast cancer and the Million Women Study. *Lancet.* 2003; **362:** 419.) (*See* **Learning point.**)

22 **Answer C:** This lady has several risk factors for post-menopausal osteoporosis, including early onset (< 45 years) menopause, absence of hormone replacement therapy, calcium and vitamin D supplementation and low body weight. Patients with osteoporosis may have no warning signs until the first fracture occurs. Gradual height loss and dorsal kyphosis may result from microfractures or complete fractures of vertebral bodies.

23 **Answer A:** Primary hyperparathyroidism remains the most common cause of hypercalcaemia in this age group. Further investigations to confirm the diagnosis would include: PTH, calcium/creatinine clearance (if < 0.01, the diagnosis is more likely to be familial hypocalciuric hypercalcaemia), parathyroid isotope scan (?hyperplasia), and ultrasound scan (?hyperplasia).

24 **Answer C:** Cushing's disease (pituitary-based hypercortisolism) fails to suppress completely after low dose dexamethasone; the high dose test is rarely done these days. Usually the cause is a basophilic adenoma.

25 **Answer A:** This man has hypogonadotrophic hypogonadism (low testosterone but LH and FSH are inappropriately low normal) indicating pituitary involvement. But, the features of this disorder in a middle aged male with a pigmented appearance, gynaecomastia and arthralgia, would suggest a diagnosis of haemochromatosis and a transferrin saturation would be the most appropriate investigation. Testes appear normal and the issue is with the pituitary so ultrasound is unnecessary (although iron deposition can also lead to primary gonadal failure). Addison's disease is not suggested by the symptoms – no weight loss mentioned, no postural features, so a short synacthen test would not be the best choice. It could be argued that pituitary MRI is appropriate as a pituitary tumour could produce these results. However, with a macroadenoma and stalk compression, prolactin may be slightly higher, visual fields may be abnormal and the arthralgia with gynaecomastia could not be explained. Finally, LH and FSH would be high in Klinefelter's syndrome, and the history also suggests that previously erectile function and development were normal.

26 **Answer B:** This patient has hypogonadotrophic hypogonadism (HH) with normal LH/FSH and low plasma total testosterone concentrations, in part due to decreased SHBG (with a relatively preserved free testosterone). HH is a relatively common scenario associated with type 2 diabetes. The exact mechanism responsible is unknown. Haemochromatosis seems unlikely in the absence of suggestive symptoms and signs (arthritis, pigmentation, hepatomegaly, deranged LFTs). Hyperprolactinaemia may be associated with HH and signs such as galactorrhoea may be present. However, as it appears that the pituitary/hypothalamic axis is not functioning properly it may be worth radiological imaging, and MRI would be the best imaging technique.

27 **Answer A:** She has subclinical hypothyroidism. The decision to treat should be based on: symptoms, positive antibodies, hypercholesterolaemia, and family history. With a TSH > 10.0, the patient is very likely to progress to overt hypothyroidism over the next ten years. In the range of 5–10, it is less clear, but if the anti-thyroid microsomal antibodies (thyroid peroxidase antibodies) are positive, the patient probably still requires treatment.

28 **Answer C:** The patient has a normal TSH and normal free T3 and T4 concentrations, excluding thyrotoxicosis, but total thyroid hormone concentrations suggest a rise in the binding globulins. This can occur in pregnancy. Sick euthyroidism would be typically associated with low thyroid hormone concentrations. Increased β-HCG in early pregnancy can lead to decreased TSH by stimulating TSH-R. This type of question can be set for both the Part I and Part II written examinations. (*See* **Learning point**.)

29 **Answer D:** Post-partum thyroiditis occurs in approximately 5% of females and is associated with transient hyperthyroidism, usually 2–6 months postpartum, followed by hypothyroidism, which also usually resolves; but permanent hypothyroidism may occur. The exact aetiology is unknown but lymphocytic infiltration of the thyroid is typical, suggesting auto-immunity through a probably similar mechanism to Hashimoto's thyroiditis. Treatment for the hyperthyroidism is usually conservative as symptoms would resolve but, if required, beta-blockers are adequate. De Quervain's thyroiditis is associated with tender enlargement of the thyroid and marked constitutional symptoms – weight loss in particular – and TFTs are often normal. A markedly elevated erythrocyte sedimentation rate would also be expected and the mild elevation in this patient may be explained by her mild anaemia.

30 **Answer A:** This patient has thyrotoxicosis and is now pregnant. Thyrotoxicosis is itself associated with poor pregnancy outcomes, with IUGR and miscarriage. Therefore thyrotoxicosis needs to be treated during pregnancy with anti-thyroid medication. The patient should be rendered euthyroid and euthyroidism should then be maintained on the lowest dose of anti-thyroid medication. A block and replacement regime is contraindicated, as both

carbimazole and propylthiouracil cross the placenta far better than thyroxine, and so may induce fetal hypothyroidism. There is little to choose between carbimazole and propylthiouracil. It was once considered that carbimazole induced aplasia cutis in the fetus, but this has more recently been disputed as aplasia cutis may be an effect of thyrotoxicosis rather than a side effect of carbimazole. Consequently, the patient should continue treatment with carbimazole. Radioactive iodine is absolutely contraindicated in pregnancy. Any surgery should be reserved for the last resort in pregnancy, as it is associated with increased risk of miscarriage. The pregnancy can progress without problems if the thyrotoxicosis is adequately treated.

# Learning Points

## Question 10

### Learning point

**Causes of hypoglycaemia**

Alcohol

Hypopituitarism, isolated ACTH deficiency, Addison's disease, sepsis

Drugs: sulphonylureas, quinine, salicylates, propanolol

Others: lung cancer, hepatoma, fulminant hepatic failure, terminal renal failure, retroperitoneal sarcoma, insulinoma, glycogen storage disorders, paediatric conditions

## Question 22

### Learning point

A *T*-score refers to the difference in standard deviation (SD) from the mean bone mass. The World Health Organization (WHO) criteria for the diagnosis of osteoporosis are as follows:

| ***T*-score** | **Normal** | **≥−1.0** |
|---|---|---|
| | Osteopaenia | −1.0 – −2.5 |
| | Osteoporosis | ≤ −2.5 |
| | Severe osteoporosis with fragility fracture | ≤ −2.5 |

## Question 28

### Learning point

Causes of an **increased** thyroid binding globulin: familial, pregnancy, oestrogen therapy, phenothiazines, hypothyroidism

Causes of a **decreased** thyroid binding globulin: familial, androgens, Cushing's disease, thyrotoxicosis, major illness, malnutrition

# Index

Note: questions and answers are given in the following format: Q/A. Learning points are given in **bold**.


ACE inhibitors
 adverse effects 38/44; 188/217–18
 contraindications 6/13
 diabetic conditions 195/221; 198/222
 regimes 5/13; 190/218–19
acoustic neuroma 239/270
acute myocardial infarction
 drug therapies 5/13
 inferior 8/13–14; 9/14
 posterior 6/13
Addison's disease 293/311; 294/311–12
adrenal failure 294/311
adrenal steroids, normal values 281
alcohol dependence syndrome 4/12
allergic rhinitis 151/168
allopurinol 116/122
aluminium toxicity 184/216
amnesia, transient global 244/272
amoebic abscesses, liver 77/85
amoebic dysentery 70/84
amyloidosis 8/14; 176/212; 184/215–16
anaemia
 MAHA (microangiopathic haemolytic) 183/214–15; **229**
 sideroblastic 29/41
aneurysm, left ventricular 2/12
angioedema
 captopril-induced 38/44
 classical hereditary 36/43
ankylosing spondylitis 92/99
anterior pituitary hormones, normal values 281–2
anthrax, lesions 51/53; 78/86
anticonvulsant therapy, and pregnancy 237/269–70
antithrombin III deficiency 201/224
aortic stenosis
 prognosis indicators 10/15
 severe 11/15
 valve replacement 11/15
ARDS (acute respiratory distress syndrome) 151/168; 154/169
ascites, treatments 140/146
aspiration 153/169
asthma
 cough-variant 166/172
 treatments 166/172–3
atrial fibrillation, drug regimes 9/14
autosomal dominant polycystic kidney disease 208–9/226–7
azathioprine 130/144; 132/145

baclofen toxicity 235/269
basilar migraine 257/275

Behcet's syndrome 92/99
bendrofluazide 193/220
benign fasciculation syndrome 260/276–7
benign intracranial hypertension 257/275; **280**
bilirubin abnormalities, post viral infections 21/39
blackwater fever 70/84
bone marrow aplasia, drug-induced 112/121
bone marrow suppression, chlorambucil therapy 32/42
botulism 242/271
bronchitis, chronic 150/168
brucellosis 66/83
bruising 23/39–40; 27/41
burn injuries 154/169

CAPRICORN trial 5/13
captopril, side effects 38/44; 187/217
carbon monoxide poisoning 109/120–1
carcinoid syndrome 139/146
cardiac failure, drug regimes 115/122
cardiology 1–16/12–15
carpal tunnel syndrome 254/274
carvedilol 5/13
cellulitis, antibiotic resistance 56/81
cerebellar haemorrhage 258/275–6
cerebral salt wasting syndrome 204/224–5
cerebrospinal fluid, normal values 233
cervical myelopathy 252/274
chemotherapy complications
    tumour lysis syndrome 31/42
    vincristine side effects 32/42
chlorambucil 32/42
chloroquine overdose 71/84
cholangitis, recurrent 143/147
cholestasis of pregnancy 128/144
cholesterol, emboli 179/213
choriocarcinoma 34/43
chronic obstructive pulmonary disease (COPD)
    acute respiratory acidosis 159/171
    characteristics 162–3/171–2
    long-term oxygen therapy 160/171
Churg-Strauss syndrome 189/218

classical hereditary angioedema 36/43
clindamycin 56/81
*Clostridium difficile* 59/82
cluster headaches 255/275
coagulation factors 17–18
coeliac disease 131/144–5
common peroneal nerve palsy 254/274
compulsive polydipsia 207/226
congenital heart problems, Jervell-Lange-Nielsen syndrome 10/14
craniopharyngioma 239/270
Creutzfeld-Jacob disease (CJD), sporadic 248/272
Crohn's disease 64/83; 130/144; 132/145
cryoglobulinaemia 37/44; 60/82
CSF lymphocytosis 259/276; **280**
Cushing's disease 302/314
cutaneous anthrax 51/53; 78/86
cystic fibrosis 167/173
cystitis 197/221–2

De Quervain's tenosynovitis 91/98
dengue haemorrhagic fever 72/84
depression, with psychosis 267/278
diabetes insipidus 206/226
diabetes mellitus
    cardiovascular risk management 288/310
    drug regimes 196/221; 197/221–2; 288/310
    nephropathy 178/213
    renal disease management 198/222
    retinopathy 195/221
dialysis patients
    amyloidosis 184/215–16
    autosomal dominant polycystic kidney disease 208/226–7
    haemoglobin levels 183/215
diffuse Lewy body disease 247/272
digoxin poisoning 106/119–20; **124**
diptheria 68/83–4
disseminated intravascular coagulation (DIC) 28/41
drug administration doses 103
dyskinesia, primary ciliary 167/173
dystonia, drug-induced 266/278
dystrophia myotonica 251/273–4

'ecstasy' abuse 105/119; **124**
ecthyma contagiosum 78/86
embolism, cholesterol 179/213
enalapril 118/123
endocrinology, normal values 281–2
eosinophilia, pulmonary 112/121
epilepsy, management during pregnancy 237/269–70
episodic paroxysmal hemicrania 256/275
essential hypertension 116/122
ethambutol-induced optic neuritis 263/277

Fabry's disease 286/309
fainting 5/13
Fallot's tetralogy 11/15
familial hyperparathyroidism 298/312–13
fasciculation syndrome 260/276–7
fibrinogen replacement infusion 28/41
fibromyalgia 95/100
fits 5/13
Fitz-Hugh-Curtis syndrome 65/83
flecainide 9/14
foot drop, common peroneal nerve palsy 254/274
fractures, pathological 24/40; 35/43; **47**
Friedreich's ataxia 251/273
frontotemporal degeneration 234/269

galactosaemia 285/308–9
gastrectomy, 'lag storage' curves 129/144
gastric carcinoma, metastatic 36/43
giant cell arteritis 94/100
*Giardia lamblia intestinalis* 56/81
Gilbert's syndrome 21/39
glaucoma, acute 262/277
gliclazide 116/122
glomerulonephropathy 200–1/223–4
gold therapy, side effects 112/121; 177/212–13
gonococcal sepsis 57/81
gout 90/98
Guillain-Barré syndrome 241/271

haematinics, normal values 18
haematology, normal values 17–19
haematuria 199/222; **229**
haemochromatosis
  hereditary (HH) 138/146
  treatments 303/314
haemoglobinuria 23/39–40
haemolytic conditions, hereditary intravascular 26/41
haemolytic uraemic syndrome (HUS) 183/214–15
haemosiderosis, pulmonary 165/172
Ham's test 23/39–40
headaches
  basilar migraine 257/275
  benign intracranial hypertension 256/275
  cluster type 255/275
  episodic paroxysmal hemicrania 256/275
heart block 9/14
heart failure, drug regimes 115/122
hemiballistic movements 236/269
hemicrania 256/275
Henoch-Schonlein purpura (HSP) 190/218–19
heparin-induced thrombocytopaenia (HIT) 30/42
hepatitis, chronic active autoimmune (CAH) 136/146
hepatitis-A 62/82; 72/84
hepatitis-B 133/145
hepatitis-C 60/82; 133/145
hereditary haemochromatosis (HH) 138/146
hereditary spherocytosis 26/41
hirudin therapy 30/42
HIV
  associated skin conditions 50/52
  visual acuity problems 263/277
HLA-B27 61/82; 92/99
HLA-DR4 94/100
Hodgkin's disease 31/42; 200/223
Holmes-Adie pupil 237/270
Horner's syndrome 238/270
HRT, and osteoporosis 93/99; 300–1/313–14
hungry bone syndrome 300/313
Huntington's disease 248/272

HUS (haemolytic uraemic syndrome) 22/39; **46**; 183/214–15
hydatid cysts 74/85
hydrocephalus 249/272
hyperbilirubinaemia 21/39
hypercalcaemia 34/43
hypercalcaemia, and hyperparathyroidism 299/313
hypernephroma 79/86
hyperparathyroidism 298/312–13; 301/314
hyperpyrexia 105/119; **124**
hypertension
  diabetic nephropathy 178/213
  IgA nephropathy 199/222
  intracranial 256/275; 257/275
  obese patients 117/122–3; 289/310
  pregnant patients 118/123
  severe and abrupt 118/123
  treatments 117/122; 118/123
  types 116/122
hypertensive nephropathy 178/213
hypertrophic obstructive cardiomyopathy 9/14
hyperviscosity syndrome 25/40–1
hypoadrenalism 292/311; 295/312
hypocalcaemia 300/313
hypoglycaemia
  Addison's disease 293/311
  insulin-induced 290/310–11
hypogonadotrophic hypogonadism (HH) 303/314; 304/315
hypothyroidism 236/269; 305/315
hypovolaemia 182/214

IgA deficiency conditions 37/44; 131/144–5
IgA nephropathy 199/222
immunology, normal values 18–19
infective endocarditis 2/12
interstitial lung disease (ILD) 161/171
interstitial nephritis 177/212–13
intravascular coagulation 28/41
intravascular haemolysis 26/41
iron treatments, in renal failure 184/215

Jervell-Lange-Nielsen syndrome 10/14
juvenile dermatomyositis (JDMS) 96/100

keratoacanthoma 51/52–3
kidney dialysis *see* dialysis patients
kidney transplants 186/216–17; 208–9/227
Kronkite-Canada syndrome 129/144

labetalol 298/312–13
lactose intolerance 283/308
'lag storage' curves 129/144
Lambert-Eaton myaesthenic syndrome 260/276
Langerhans' cell histriocytosis 164/172
lansoprazole 116/122
laxative abuse 283/308
Leber's optic atrophy 261/277
left ventricular aneurysm 2/12
legionnaire's disease 76/85; 80/86
leishmaniasis 68/83
leptospirosis 62/82; 63/82
leucocyte enzymes, normal values 282
Lewy body disease 247/272
lipids, normal values 282
lipoproteins, normal values 282
lisinopril 116/122
listeria 74/85
lithium toxicity 104/119; 111/121
liver
  amoebic abscesses 77/85
  non-alcoholic fatty liver disease (NAFLD) 137/146
Lofgren's syndrome 150/168
long QT syndrome 10/14–15; **16**
loss of consciousness 5/13
low back pain, red flags 96/100
lung cancer, squamous cell carcinoma 152/169; 155/170
lung collapse 153/169
lung disease, interstitial sclerosis-associated 161/171
lung fibrosis 96/100; 158/170–1
lupus pernio 150/168
Lyme disease 58/81–2; 62/82; 240/271

MAHA (microangiopathic haemolytic anaemia) 183/214–15; **229**
malaria 67/83; 70/84
*Malassezia* yeast infections 50/52

malignant melanomas 51/53
membraneous glomerulonephritis 201/223–4
meningitis
  bacterial 75/85
  investigations 259/276
  treatments 59/82; 75/85
mesothelioma 151/168
metformin 116/122
methaemoglobinaemia 157/170
methanol ingestion 107–8/120
methyldopa 118/123
metoclopramide, overdose 266/278
microangiopathic haemolytic anaemia (MAHA) 22/39; **46**
migraine, basilar 257/275
motor neurone disease 250/273
MTU/MTT 34/43
multiple endocrine neoplasia (MEN) type-1 297/312; 298/312
multiple endocrine neoplasia (MEN) type-2 298/312
multiple sclerosis 261/277
multiple system atrophy 245/272
muscle twitching 250/273; 260/276–7
myaesthenia gravis 243/271–2
*Mycoplasma pneumoniae* 156/170
myeloma 24/40; 35/43
myocardial infarction
  drug therapies 5/13
  inferior 8/13–14; 9/14
  posterior 6/13
myositis, juvenile dermatomyositis (JDMS) 96/100
myotonic dystrophy (MD) 251/273–4

necrotising fasciitis 63/82
nephrology, normal values 175
nephrotic syndrome, management 176/212; 203/224
neuralgic amyotrophy 252/274
neurofibromatosis type-1 50/52
neuroleptic malignant syndrome (NMS) 268/278
neutropenia
  causes **125**
  sulphasalazine-induced 113/121; **125**
non-alcoholic fatty liver disease (NAFLD) 137/146
non-seminomatous germ cell tumours (NSGCTs) 35/43
nose bleeds 25/40–1; 27/41
NSAIDs, side effects 177/212–13

obesity
  diabetes and cardiovascular risk 289/310
  and hypertension 117/122–3; 202/224; 289/310
  hypertriglyceridaemia 311/291
ocreotide 139/146
oestrogen therapy 93/99
oliguria 182/214
omeprazole 115/122
optic atrophy 261–2/277
optic neuritis 263/277
orbital apex syndrome 240/271
orf 78/86
osmotic fragility studies 26/41
osteoarthritis, hands 91/98
osteomalacia 111/121
osteomyelitis 185/216
osteoporosis 93/99; 300–1/313–14; **317**
oxygen therapy
  long-term use 150/168; 160/171
  positive pressure ventilation 159/171

pacing
  perforation (ventricular rupture) 8/13–14
  permanent 9/14
  temporary 9/14
Paget's disease 97/100–1
pamidronate 34/43; 35/43
pancreatic hormones, normal values 282
paracetamol, overdose 104/119
parathyroid carcinoma 296/312
parkinsonian syndrome 245/272
Parkinson's disease, tremor management 249/273
paroxysmal nocturnal haemoglobinuria 23/39–40
parvovirus B19 infection 95/100; **102**
patent foramen ovale 3/12

peritonitis, spontaneous bacterial 141/147
peroneal nerve palsy 254/274
pharmacology, therapeutic drug levels 103
phenothiazine, side effects 110/121
phenytoin
  therapy 111/121
  toxicity 105/119
pityriasis rosea 51/52
pityriasis versicolor 50/52
pneumonia
  atypical 88
  community-acquired 153/169
  gram-negative bacteria 80/86
  *Legionella* infections 80/86
  *Mycoplasma* infections 156/170
  prognosis indicators 153/169
polyarteritis nodosa 37/44
polycystic kidney disease 208–9/226–7
polycystic ovary syndrome (PCOS) 285/309
polydipsia 207/226
porphyria, acute intermittent 284/308
portal hypertension 132/145; **148**
portal vein thrombosis 132/145
pregnancy
  cholestasis 128/144
  hypertension 118/123
  thyroid hormones 305–7/315–16; **317**
  Wernicke's encephalopathy 265/278
primary ciliary dyskinesia 167/173
pseudofits 5/13
psoriasis, drug-induced complications 51/53
psoriatic arthritis 93/99
pulmonary embolism, risk factors 152/169
pulmonary eosinophilia 112/121
pulmonary fibrosis 96/100; 158/170–1
pulmonary haemosiderosis 165/172
purpuric rashes
  cryoglobulinaemia 37/44
  Henoch-Schonlein purpura (HSP) 190/218–19
  heparin-induced thrombocytopaenia (HIT) 30/42
  hepatitis-C 60/82
  TTP (thrombotic thrombocytopaenic purpura) 22/39; **46**
pyogenic granuloma 51/52–3

Q fever 73/84–5

radiculopathy 253/274
ramipril 176/212
reflux nephropathy 191/219; 192/219–20
reinfarction 8/13–14
Reiter's syndrome 57/81; 58/81–2
renal calculi 193–4/220–1
renal failure
  hyperuricaemic nephropathy 31/42
  iron treatments 184/215
  NSAID-induced 177/212–13
  treatments 181/214
renal infarction 7/13
renal transplant 186/216–17; 208–9/227
respiratory distress syndrome, acute 151/168; 154/169
restless leg syndrome 250/273
rhabdomyolysis 114/121–2; 211/228; **231**
rheumatoid arthritis, prognostic indicators 94/100
rheumatology, normal values 18–19, 89
risedronate 300/313–14
Rocky Mountain spotted fever 62/82

sacral plexopathy 255/275
salmeterol 166/172–3
sarcoidosis 132/145; 150/168; **174**; 154/170
schistosomiasis 69/84
schizophrenia
  characteristics 264/277
  neuroleptic malignant syndrome (NMS) 268/278
scurvy 287/309–10
seborrhoeic eczema 50/52
selective IgA deficiency 37/44
septicaemia, treatments 181/214
serotonin syndrome 210/227–8
sex hormones, normal values 282
shooting pains 253/274
SIADH (syndrome of inappropriate ADH) 205/225; **230**

sickle cell disorders 20/39; **45**; 199/222
sideroblastic anaemia 29/41
simvastatin, side effects 114/121–2
smoking cessation 152/168
sodium valproate 237/269–70
spherocytosis 26/41
spironolactone 140/146
squamous cell carcinoma, bronchogenic 152/169; 155/170
staphylococcal arthritis 58/81–2
Still's disease 96/100; **102**
*Streptococci* infections, antibiotic resistance 56/81
stroke
  DVT and PFO 3/12
  hemiballistic movements 236/269
subthalamic nucleus lesions 236/269
sulphasalazine therapy, side effects 113/121
superior vena caval obstruction (SVCO) 33/42–3
synacthen test 293–5/311–12
syncope 5/13; 11/15
syphilis, neonates 67/83
syringomyelia 251/273
systemic lupus erythematosus 180/213–14
systemic sclerosis 118/123
systemic vasculitis 37/44

*T*-scores **317**
testicular tumours 35/43; 46–7
tetracycline, side effects 112/121
thiamine deficiency 4/12
thiazide diuretics 117/122
thrombus, intra-cardiac 7/13
thyroid hormones
  normal values 282
  and pregnancy 305–6/315; **317**
thyroiditis, post-partum 306/315
thyrotoxicosis 307/315–16
transient global amnesia 244/272
transient ischaemic attacks (TIAs) 258/276
transplant rejection, renal 186/216–17
tricyclic antidepressants (TCAs), overdose 110/121
TTP (thrombotic thrombocytopaenic purpura) 22/39; **46**
tuberculous arthritis 58/81–2; 90/98
tuberculous ileitis 64/83
tumour lysis syndrome 31/42
twitching 250/273; 260/276–7
typhoid 70/84

ulnar neuropathy, elbow 253/274
ureteric reflux 191/219
urinary tract infections 191–2/219–20
urine, normal values 282

vasculitis, systemic 37/44
ventricular rupture, pacing wire perforation 8/13–14
vertebral artery dissection 239/270; 279–80
vesicoureteric reflux (VUR) 191–2/219–20
vincristine 32/42
vision loss
  acute glaucoma 262/277
  unilateral 25/40–1
von Willebrand disease 27/41

Waldenstrom's macroglobulinaemia 25/40–1
Wallenburg's syndrome 238/270
Wernicke's encephalopathy 265–6/278
Whipple's disease 61/82
Wilson's disease 135/145

yellow fever 72/84

zolendronic acid 34/43